Arts Therapies and Progressive Illness

Arts Therapies and Progressive Illness is a guide to the use of arts therapies in the treatment of patients with diseases such as Parkinson's and Alzheimer's. In the last few years arts therapies have been used in an increasingly wide range of applications with new groups of patients, such as patients in palliative care, or with learning disabilities – Diane Waller has been a driving force behind this expansion.

This book covers treatments such as art therapy, dance movement therapy and music therapy. In addition to dealing with a wide range of debilitating diseases, it focuses on the issue of the care and treatment of dementia and the effects on patients, carers and staff and the role of the arts therapies in improving the quality of life for the increasing number of patients who will sadly develop this distressing illness.

The broadly focused, multi-disciplinary book will be of great interest to arts therapists, arts therapy educators, medial, social work and other staff who are concerned to devise care plans for these patients and their relatives.

Diane Waller is Professor of Art Therapy at Goldsmiths College. Her previous publications include *Becoming a Profession: the History of Art Therapy in Britain 1940–82* (1991), *Group-Interactive Art Therapy* (1993) and *Treatment of Addiction* (1998, co-edited with Jacqueline Mahony).

Arts Therapies and Progressive Illness

Nameless Dread

Edited by Diane Waller

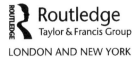

Routledge
Taylor & Francis Group

LONDON AND NEW YORK

First published 2002 by Routledge
27 Church Road, Hove, East Sussex BN3 2FA

Simultaneously published in the USA and Canada
by Routledge
270 Madison Ave, New York NY 10016

Routledge is an imprint of the Taylor & Francis Group, an informa business

Transferred to Digital Printing 2010

Typeset in Times by RefineCatch Limited, Bungay, Suffolk

Paperback cover design by Terry Foley
Paperback cover illustration from a painting by Daniel Lumley,
entitled 'Parkinson's Disease', made shortly after he received a
diagnosis of Parkinson's.

British Library Cataloguing in Publication Data
A catalogue record for this book is available from the British Library

Library of Congress Cataloging in Publication Data
Arts therapies and progressive illness : nameless dread / edited by
   Diane Waller.
      p. cm.
   Includes bibliographical references and index.
   ISBN 0–415–21980–9—ISBN 0–415–21981–7 (pbk.)
   1. Art therapy. 2. Arts—Therapeutic use. 3. Dementia—
Patients—Care. 4. Alzheimer's disease—Patients—Care.
   I. Waller, Diane.
   RC489.A72 A775 2002
   615.8'5156—dc21   2002025439

ISBN 978–0–415–21981–5 (pbk)

Publisher's Note
The publisher has gone to great lengths to ensure the quality of this reprint
but points out that some imperfections in the original may be apparent.

Like one, that on a lonesome road
Doth walk in fear and dread,
And having once turned round walks on
And turns no more his head;
Because he knows a frightful fiend
Doth close behind him tread.

Coleridge,
The Rime of the Ancient Mariner

Contents

List of contributors   ix
Foreword by Robin Higgins   xiii
Acknowledgements   xv

1 Arts therapies, progressive illness, dementia: the difficulty of being   1
   DIANE WALLER

2 In the waiting room of the Grim Reaper   13
   KEN EVANS

3 The living death: dance movement therapy with Parkinson's
   patients   27
   JILL BUNCE

4 Art therapy in the treatment of chronic invalidating conditions:
   from Parkinson's disease to Alzheimer's   47
   ATTILIA COSSIO

5 Case studies in Huntington's disease: music therapy assessment
   and treatment in the early to advanced stages   56
   WENDY L. MAGEE

6 Art therapy with older adults clinically diagnosed as having
   Alzheimer's disease and dementia   68
   JOHN TYLER

7 Real world or fantasy?   84
   KEN EVANS

8   Living with dementia: interview with Neil McArthur   94
    DIANE WALLER

9   A narrowed sense of space: an art therapy group with young
    Alzheimer's sufferers   107
    BARRY FALK

10 Evaluating the use of art therapy for older people with
    dementia: a control group study   122
    DIANE WALLER

    Case vignette: FINLAY MCINALLY   134

11 Changing the context of care: opening up the system; interview
    with Kamal Beeharee   138
    DIANE WALLER

12 Art as a therapy for Parkinson's   145
    NANCY TINGEY

13 Circles of the mind: the use of therapeutic circle dance with
    older people with dementia   165
    DOROTHY JERROME

14 Nameless dread: a carer's story   183
    DIANE WALLER

Index   195

Contributors

Kamal Beeharee is a registered mental nurse with a background in therapeutic management. He is co-ordinator of services for people with early onset dementia in Brighton and Hove and has extensive experience with elderly mentally ill and older patients with dementia. He is now manager of the Towner Club, which is a day club for younger people with dementia. Kamal is committed to patient-led and therapeutic community models when providing services for people with mental illness and/or dementia.

Jill Bunce is a dance movement therapist whose MA at the Laban Centre focused on DMT with Parkinson's patients. Jill lectures in universities in the UK and abroad, linking the theory and practice of neuroscience with psychoanalysis, child development and learning difficulties. She was made an honorary member of the neurological department of Staffordshire General Infirmary, and is now establishing research work into palliative care in the arts therapies, particularly in the area of degenerative illness, dementia and care of the dying. Her current practice is with people with multiple sclerosis, Parkinson's disease and children with autism, learning difficulties and disabilities.

Attilia Cossio is a teacher of drawing and history of art as well as an art therapist. She was driven towards art therapy by a personal need for research on the basis of her work as a teacher. She was trained at Il Porto (ADEG) in Turin, Italy. At present she trains staff and leads art therapy groups with adults and elderly people, developing support systems for different pathologies. With Vera Zilzer she published *L'Ombrello a colori. Metodi, case ed esperienze di arte-terapia* (Franco Angeli, 1997).

Ken Evans combines his academic and professional interests in working as a consultant and as a lecturer in social policy and social sciences, contributing to the psychotherapy programmes at Goldsmiths College. After graduating in Philosophy at London, he took a B.Sc. in Sociology and Psychology at Bristol, followed by an MA in Social Theory and a D.Phil. at the University of Santa Tomas, Philippines. He is a Fellow of the Royal

Anthropological Society and has conducted research in mental health, elderly care, education and training for social work. His current interests are in combining and integrating theoretical perspectives from all fields of human traditions and categories in the application of care.

Barry Falk is an artist and art therapist. While training at Goldsmiths College he was awarded the Corinne Burton Scholarship, enabling him to specialise in work with cancer patients or those with terminal illnesses. He currently runs an art therapy group on the Oncology Ward of the Royal Sussex Hospital, at the Towner Club, Martlets Hospice and at two of the centres featured in the Apollo Art Therapy Research Project in Brighton and Newhaven.

Dorothy Jerrome spent nearly 25 years in higher education as a social gerontologist at the universities of Sussex and Southampton before moving on to Age Concern in Brighton, Hove and Portslade. She currently works as a training and development officer in older people's services in local government. Her chapter draws together her knowledge of the ageing person and the existential world of dementia, her love of dance and belief in its transformative capacity.

Neil McArthur was academic registrar at King's College, London before moving into work with the Alzheimer's Society in Brighton. He is now the manager of the Brighton and Hove branch, developing an extensive network of volunteers who give respite to relatives of people with dementia and providing training. Neil was instrumental in setting up the research project on the needs of people with early onset dementia and their carers, and in bringing the Towner Club into existence.

Wendy L. Magee is a music therapist clinician, researcher and manager at the Royal Hospital for Neuro-disability in London. She trained at the University of Melbourne, Australia before coming to work in London. She has worked in the field of neurology for about 12 years. She completed doctoral research on comparing song and improvisation with individuals with chronic neurological illness. Wendy is visiting tutor for the foundation Music Therapy programme at Goldsmiths College, London.

Finlay McInally is an artist and art therapist, trained at Goldsmiths College, now specialising in work with the elderly and severely psychotic patients. He was the art therapist in the Pilot Art Therapy Research project conducted prior to the Apollo Project, and is now running two groups for the latter, as well as working in South Downs Trust with adult mentally ill patients.

Nancy Tingey is an artist, art curator and adult education teacher. In 1994 she founded Painting with Parkinson's, an art group for people with PD and their carers, in Canberra, Australia. Nancy combined her role as a carer for her husband with PD with her art education background and in 1996 she was awarded a Churchill Fellowship, enabling her to travel extensively to study art as therapy for PD. She developed a specialised art programme for PD which has become a role model for others. Since returning to the UK in 1999 she has run workshops for Young Onset Parkinson's, Partners and Relatives and the Parkinson's Information Network, organised conferences and tutored for the Parkinson's Disease Society 'Art for Parkinson's' pilot trial.

John Tyler came to art therapy with a background of art teaching in primary through to secondary level. While training as an art therapist at Goldsmiths he did a placement with older adults and later went on to develop his work with older people with dementia, using both group and individual approaches. John recently completed a psychotherapy training and is now exploring the hypothesis that art therapy can assist people experiencing memory loss to resolve significant conflicts during the final stages of their lives. He is Head Art Therapist in an NHS Trust hospital in Surrey.

Diane Waller founded the Art Psychotherapy Unit at Goldsmiths College, London. She is Professor of Art Therapy there, and Visiting Professor in the School of Psychology at Queen's University, Belfast and at Brighton University. Her research has included the history and development of the profession of art therapy in the UK and abroad, action research on art therapy training, art therapy with eating disorders, groups, drug addiction, and currently with older people with dementia. Her background in art, ethnography, dance and the process model of sociology has led her to question many of the assumptions prevalent in the 'caring' professions. This was heightened by her experience of being 'carer' for her husband with Parkinson's related dementia.

Foreword
Robin Higgins

By a number of measures, this is an important and wide-ranging book. Ostensibly about dementia and the contribution that arts therapists can make to relieving the 'nameless dread' that lies behind dementia's implacable tread, a cursory reading will quickly reveal that topics broached extend far beyond these limits.

In the first place, the population of those suffering from dementia must be a key issue in any society that has to cope with increasing longevity. Whom now do we class as elderly? Several case studies in this book describe people who are in their forties and fifties, with the prospect of many more years ahead of them, depending on a set of interrelated issues: physical health; a sense of identity, place, and purpose; the retained capacity for enjoyment.

An equally glaring point, dementia is not confined to those who suffer from it themselves. There are those designated officially and somehow inadequately as the carers, both among the relatives, spouses, and friends, and among the care homes and hospital staff, all of whom are drawn into this engulfing circle of need. Several chapters in the book are given over to poignant descriptions of what is entailed in becoming entangled in the web of dementia: from bearing witness to the slow dissolution of a loved one (as John Bayley bore for Iris Murdoch) to disentangling the confusions of projective identifications. Other chapters outline some of the management problems that give rise to institutional paradoxes. Among many examples cited, two situations stand out: one where personal care and concern, the lifelines for someone in the throes of dementia, and the very purpose for which the institution was set up, become threatened or destroyed by rigid routines; the other where sustained atmospheres of 'hysterical merriment' are imposed to jolly carers and patients alike out of their all too understandable moments of authentic and healing sadness.

So in the second place, the book faces us with some stark questions. What are we expecting of carers, whether family, friends, or staff? And what sort of support are we providing them with in their acutely difficult task of fulfilling these expectations? In a cultural ethic where great emphasis is placed on market values, and winning (from league tables to the most up-to-date weaponry), where to advance up a career ladder we appear to need increasing specialisation and segmentation (witness the medical and sociological networks spelt out in Ken Evans's chapters), what time can we really spare for those whom dementia and related progressive debilities have sidelined?

The issue takes us far beyond the sphere of politicians and economic planners, where we have often been only too happy to dump it. It devolves on the question of understanding the other-in-the-margin, and that is one of the questions on which the whole future of our species depends.

The third reason why this book is important are the glimpses it offers of a landscape with some exciting possibilities. These go along with a number of sea-changes which are occurring in the scientific and humanities background and of which arts therapists are well placed to take advantage.

Neurological and biochemical studies, for example, are opening up our understanding of how physical forces link with psychological and social ones in psyche-soma networks that ramify (as Freud and others intuited) well below the 5 per cent of mental activity we call 'conscious'. We're moving to a position where a state like dementia can no longer be dismissed as 'just organic', since we know now that organic is not only linked through field forces to the inorganic but also through emotive channels to the realm of ideational expression.

One doesn't have to be a dancer or a singer (though it sometimes helps) to appreciate the subtleties implicit in the physical postures we assume every moment of our lives and of which we are usually quite unaware. The ideas they convey to us and to others – the body language – may lead to our walking on air, or falling in the ditch in a knot. In her chapter on Parkinson's, Jill Bunce singles out posture as just one body–mind–spirit expression which has infinite potential and with which an arts therapist can hold a non-verbal dialogue with the patient. Dorothy Jerrome elaborates similar possibilities inherent in the touch and rhythms of circular dance.

The confluence of the neurosciences and psychoanalysis, and of trance, hypnosis, and visualisation must be grist to the arts therapists' mill, since so much of their work occurs at a non-verbal or pre-verbal level, and they do not feel compelled to move prematurely from a procedural (the drawing, the improvisation, the gesture) to a declarative symbol, verbalising what it's all about. Of course, this move from procedural to declarative may happen, but when it does, as John Tyler observes, something is laid to rest in a different way than if words only were used.

Another complementary polarity addressed in the book is that between narrative-based and evidence-based approaches. Two detailed control group studies (Diane Waller's and Dorothy Jerrome's) offer a valuable counterweight to the many lively narratives of dramatic events that bring a scene and a person to life. This balance of science and humanity informs and illustrates the book's endeavour: creative understanding to improve the quality of life.

Acknowledgements

There are many people who have made this book possible as a result of their goodwill and support. The first acknowledgement must go to the contributors themselves. I would also like to mention in particular Mary and John Bean, Celia Young, Neil McArthur and the volunteers from the Alzheimer's Society, Kamal Beeharee and Ray Watkinson. Thanks go also to colleagues at Routledge, especially to Kate Hawes and Dominic Hammond.

The book is dedicated to the late Daniel Lumley and Ilya Sabev, to Maria Sabev, and to all the known and unknown sufferers from progressive illness and their carers.

Chapter 1

Arts therapies, progressive illness, dementia

The difficulty of being

Diane Waller

Art therapists have traditionally worked with patients excluded from verbal psychotherapy services, beginning in the 1940s and 1950s with so-called 'chronically mentally ill' or 'burnt out' patients, later in the 1970s with the 'severely mentally handicapped' and in the past two decades with elderly dementing patients. As early as the 1860s, asylums housing chronically ill, psychotic patients and those suffering from 'senile dementia' were providing arts activities, but not all had access to the 'entertainment' they provided and the preferred option for such patients was work (Skailes, 1997: 199).

The results of encouraging patients with virtually no verbal communication, who were severely depressed and isolated, and for whom hope had been lost, to engage in visual, musical or bodily expression were often startlingly positive (Wood, 1997: 144–175; Henzell, 1997: 176–197). Although access to the arts was on a very *ad hoc* basis, the beneficial effects of 'arts therapy' on these extremely withdrawn people led some prominent medical practitioners to support the development of the arts therapies as effective interventions.[1] Despite the growing number of reputable arts therapy publications focusing on specialised client groups, many of the positive effects of these therapies with people suffering from progressive or degenerative illnesses remain undocumented, known only to recipients, carers and the immediate health care team. Systematic research, from detailed case work to control group studies, is urgently needed to remedy this situation.

Although not all progressive illnesses lead to dementia, there are many that do, including stroke, Parkinson's (and its variants), Alzheimer's and Huntington's disease. Dementia is described as a condition which involves a severe decline in an individual's mental abilities, most markedly in language, judgement, reasoning and memory (Terry and Katzman, 1992). One of the major effects of a dementing illness is the concomitant emergence of depression, one of the effects of which is a reduced cognitive capability. The impact of a diagnosis of dementia on the sufferer and their family and friends is often underestimated. It is a sentence of 'no hope', condemning all concerned to a never-ending series of losses and humiliations. The terms 'progressive illness' and 'organic brain disorder' bring with them suggestions of rapid, unrelieved deterioration, and it is not surprising to find that the sufferer and their relatives get very depressed, very quickly.

The arts therapies are 'person centred' and, importantly, build on the positive attributes of patients, assuming that all can be creative at some level. The materials and methods of the arts therapist are flexible, and a skilled therapist assesses the patient's capabilities, gently encouraging and supporting even the smallest mark, sound or movement. For people with dementia who have lost their identity, feel frightened in a confusing and controlling world and who can no longer express themselves through speech, writing or even perhaps touch, having access to the safe, quiet spaces of the art therapy studio, with the full attention of the therapist, can give a purpose, containment and means of being in control. This last point is very important as it may be that the person has lost control of their bodily functions as well as their emotional life and relationships. This brings a strong sense of shame and constant anxiety.

Depression, loneliness and terrible fear are features of progressive illnesses, especially of dementia. The term 'nameless dread' was chosen for the book because the person is frightened but does not know why. Bion (1957: 105) used this term in reference to the effects on a baby who constantly cries but is not answered, thus it gets terrified because obviously it is totally dependent on the adult for its survival. When the mother (or carer) does not respond to the baby's frantic crying then the baby's sense of abandonment is not dealt with. The baby's experience is that its terror cannot be managed, it cannot be comforted, and there is no safety. The fear is all-pervasive, particularly during the night (darkness, alone). A person with severe dementia, I would say, is often in a similar position to the baby, feeling abandoned in a state of terror, and it is essential that a way is found for such torment to be expressed and acknowledged.

Valerie Sinason (1992), although writing about 'mental handicap', discusses with great sensitivity many issues very relevant to people with progressive illness and dementia. Her work is very important in demonstrating that persons traditionally excluded from psychodynamic therapies, such as those with mental handicap, psychosis, dementia, may, in fact, benefit greatly from sensitive interventions. Sinason is a psychoanalytic psychotherapist working at the Tavistock Clinic and she is also a poet. Her papers and case studies are accompanied by the poems she writes to help her to manage the often painful and puzzling material of her clients. She pays great attention to the subtleties of communication, verbal and non-verbal, describing, for example, an incident when a profoundly handicapped man pours his breakfast cereal all over the table but manages to miss the cereal bowl. The residential worker confesses to feeling angry, then guilty, preferring to see this as an accident rather than a meaningful communication. The task has, however, been mismanaged with great accuracy. We may refer to such an action as 'being stupid', but Sinason points out that 'To be stupid is to be numbed with grief and those who bear the burden of a mental handicap carry an enormous amount of grief' (1992: 31). We could say the same about the persons who are the focus of this book, who by losing their memories, their faculties and their relationships, often appear 'stupid' to themselves and others.

Sinason points out that the emotional experience of the individual with late-onset physical illness or handicap is very similar to that of the mentally handicapped individual. In 'The man who was losing his brain' (1992: 87–110) Sinason writes:

> The difference between someone at the start of Alzheimer's disease and someone near the end is as large as the difference between someone who is normal and someone who is profoundly handicapped. The total continuum is experienced in the mind and heart of a single being.
>
> (1992: 89)

She describes her work with a 56-year-old man, a university lecturer when he developed Alzheimer's. She arranged to see him in his own home and continued for a year. The story is deeply moving. At one point the session was so painful that Sinason tried to encompass her experience in a poem before writing up her notes. One day she arrived at his house:

> I stood on the doorstep feeling equally lost. 'I am Mrs Sinason', I finally managed to say: 'Have you forgotten my face?' It was somehow easier to say that than to ask 'Have you forgotten me?' In feeling the experience of being lost to memory, wiped out, even momentarily, I was experiencing just a tiny moment of what Edward Johnson had to live with.
>
> (1992: 109)

Eventually Mr Johnson found the sessions too difficult: 'He found thinking harder and preferred gardening.' One year later he died. Sinason concludes:

> He had held onto thinking, as represented by my presence, as long as he could. According to his sons, therapy allowed him to come to terms with his degeneration, with the unpicking of the fine embroidery that had been his brain. However, once it got to the point of the last unravelling, when he knew mindlessness and death lay ahead, he felt better equipped to go with nature (the tree) and his mother (the scarf) and his father (the book).
>
> (1992: 110)

How to hold on to one's faculties as long as possible becomes a real challenge in organic, progressive illness and it is here that we may see some chance for the arts therapies. Visual image-making activates a part of the brain still intact, as we can observe throughout detailed analyses of art therapy case studies. Dance, music and movement provide valuable expressive and socialising possibilities and may help to reorientate the sufferer in the world. The drama of dementia is always present and although dramatherapy is not specifically addressed in this book, we may find that important elements of dramatherapy emerge in the art therapy or dance and dance movement therapy groups.

Unfortunately, very few patients with progressive illness currently have access either to psychodynamic therapy or to the arts or arts therapies. This is mainly due to the fact that many hospitals and centres catering for the elderly, who form the largest group of sufferers, do not employ an arts therapist; partly, though, it is because few doctors, and indeed few sufferers themselves, would think that it might help. Nursing homes, which house more severely dementing residents, are ill-equipped to provide spaces where creative activity can take place. There are many negative attitudes to be overcome about making a mess, fear of things getting out of control, anxiety about the use of art materials both among residents and staff. Moreover, the all-pervasive sense that 'it is no use, it is too late' has to be overcome.

The following quotes (referring to chronic psychotic patients) which I have borrowed from Salomon Resnik seem to express this well:

> Space and 'madness' are two aspects of being with which I have been concerned for a long time. What does it mean to be an individual? What does it mean to be in the world and what about the world itself? A being is not a thing, not merely an object, but mainly a subject. Being a subject, to be one's self, to be a person means to have a 'living body', a moving body, a thinking body. To be means to have a place of one's own, to experience one's body and mind as a living element in space and time. To live means to experience time ('temps vecu' in Bergson's view) and the passing of time (becoming) as part of existence . . .
>
> (1992: 221)

and he continues:

> Bion used to speak of 'wandering thoughts' searching for a thinker (or wild thoughts in search of somebody able to tame them, of someone able to contain them, to stand and understand them). The main problem in counter-transference with psychotic patients is to tolerate madness and at the same time to protect one's self from being seduced or possessed by these very thoughts . . .
>
> (1992: 222)

These images are powerful and in my experience, as well as bearing in mind Sinason's comparisons with mentally handicapped persons, we could substitute the 'person with dementia' for 'the person with a psychosis' – not in a manner designed to negate the difference in these conditions but because when one's senses, one's perceptions, one's relationships are jumbled, confused and undifferentiated this is indeed a state of madness into which those closest to the sufferer may also be drawn. It becomes urgent to find a way to reinforce a sense of self. Schaverien puts it well:

> It is through actions and symbolic forms, such as art and language, that a sense of self, and of agency, develops . . . Belonging to a group involves shared rituals and a common language: it is through these that membership of a community is confirmed. The psychotic patient suffers because he/she does not experience him/herself as a member of a community. The use of symbolic forms fails and there is no communal understanding. The spoken word cannot be relied upon to mediate. At this point pictures may form a bridge between unmediated experiences and the Other . . .
>
> (1997: 17)

Even if dementia is not present, or not yet present, there are few who can tolerate a relentless progressive loss of their faculties, an inability to feel part of the world, such an assault on their person, without feeling, at least some of the time, that they are going mad.

Thanks to the work of pioneers like Tom Kitwood between 1987 and his untimely recent death, and especially to his (1997) *Dementia Reconsidered: The Person Comes First*, and of Bère M.L. Miesen's work between 1992 and 1999, more attention is gradually being given to the possibility that people with dementia may be able to live a more fulfilling life than had hitherto seemed possible. At the time of writing this book, the English government's medicines-rationing body NICE has announced that the new and still controversial drug Aricept, and its equivalents Exelon and Reminyl, is to be made available nationwide to people with mild to moderate Alzheimer's, at an apparent cost of £45 million annually. This drug may slow the progress of deterioration for a period. Another potentially helpful vaccine, AN 1792, is currently being tested on mice, but although human trials are underway it is likely to be 3–5 years before a treatment emerges. As Neil McArthur mentions in his interview (see Chapter 8, p. 94), for the first time the possibility exists for alleviating the disease. There are many developments in the treatment of Parkinson's: in terms of dopamine (L-Dopa), which works on the neuroreceptors in the brain, and, from January 2001, in embryo research – a very controversial step but one which may produce benefits for this client group.

Perhaps the most striking point, an obvious one but often overlooked, to be made by Kitwood and other 'radical' workers is that each person with dementia is an individual, and that each person's needs are going to be different. That this should be a radical suggestion is indeed astonishing and is indicative of a socio-cultural context which is completely hypocritical in emphasising the rights of the individual but not, apparently, those of the person with dementia – especially those who are old (the majority), poor and do not have a supportive family.

This book does not pretend to provide solutions for the care and treatment of people with the grave and life-sapping illnesses discussed. It asks the question, why are things the way they are, and what might we try to do about them? It offers some positive possibilities in terms of art as therapy, and art psychotherapies. Living and working with someone who knows that the life they took for granted is gradually disappearing, that they may be physically and mentally declining but they do not know how long this will go on for, and that the outcome will be that they will be totally dependent on others, is hard in itself. Living in environments where they watch others deteriorate and disappear, and know that is probably going to be their fate, is hellish. The book will reflect the struggle of its authors (including its editor) in their efforts to come to terms with such a reality. For example, in Chapter 14 I give a personal account of my own extreme difficulty in reconciling myself to the awfulness of my late husband's condition, my own 'nameless dread', in the form of learned anxiety and panic, which even three years after his death is regularly present.

It is not only close relatives and carers of the person with progressive illness who are affected. The staff caring for the sufferer and the institutions in which they find themselves are subject to the unrelenting process of 'projective identification' (Segal 1975: 126), further confusing and distressing everyone concerned. For those unfamiliar with the term, it was coined by Melanie Klein and is defined as:

> the result of the projection of parts of the self into an object. It may result in the object being perceived as having acquired the characteristics of the projected part of the self but it can also result in the self becoming identified with the object of its projection.
>
> (Segal, 1975: 126)

In other words, such a process can lead to the other person taking on and 'acting out' the projections, which could lead to a carer getting overwhelmed by feelings of rage, hopelessness and incompetence, which are actually felt but cannot be dealt with by the person with dementia and thus projected out.

While emphasising the importance of the arts and arts therapies for patients, we also have to recognise their limitations and not assume that they are always a means of communication. Killick (1997: 40–41) usefully draws our attention to the need to recognise when a patient is making art (or mark-making) to defend themselves against unbearable anxiety and when they are trying to communicate. In the first instance Killick, drawing on Bion (1957), suggests that the art is: 'used by the patient experiencing catastrophic anxiety as a means of intrusive identification, i.e. as a way of forcibly evacuating unbearable anxieties into the art object, and that accordingly it holds evacuated beta elements' (1997: 42). She considers that patients in this state benefit from the 'concreteness of the substances and objects available to and made by the patient in the art psychotherapy setting', allowing the 'violences of the intrusive identifications to be absorbed without damage to the patient or the therapist' (1997: 43). If the therapist can tolerate the period of intrusive identification, it may be that the patient will reach a stage where they can communicate, or may make a piece of art that has the potential for communication (1997: 44). To reach such a stage will require consistent, safe, boundaried time and space and the regular presence of the therapist. As we shall see from the contributions to this book, the possibility of encountering such a desirable intervention is extremely rare for patients suffering from progressive illness and dementia.

Staff in institutions caring for people with the progressive illnesses featured in this book are, then, subject to massive projective identification which can be dangerous both for the staff and the patients, even leading to cases of abuse. Yet we find a noticeable absence of therapeutically trained employees, agency staff who come and go, minimal or no support and supervision. Surely this is one of the most difficult areas of work, being with people who have 'no hope'?

Kitwood discusses 'the nature of empathy and projective and empathetic identification' (1997: 128–130) and shows how it can happen that all kinds of difficulties may arise in a relationship with someone with dementia:

> When we develop empathy with someone who has all their mental powers intact, we attend both to their words and to their non-verbal signals. Sometimes we notice discrepancies between the two kinds of message. A person might, for example, claim to be feeling 'perfectly OK', while showing clear signs of anxiety or inner turmoil. Gradually, keeping all the information in a kind of 'soft focus' we gain a sense of what they might be experiencing.
>
> (1997: 128)

Consider, though, what happens when a caregiver gets caught up in a process of projective identification, when the caregiver will:

> 'see' aspects of his or her own self in the person who has dementia, and may even induce that person to act some of these aspects out; making them become more angry, more helpless, more confused etc.
>
> (1997: 128–129)

So, if these processes operate between the person with dementia and their relative, they obviously can do so in formal care, and it is the opinion of Kitwood, and certainly of the authors in this book, that these processes may become (in Kitwood's words) 'noxious'. When we think of the thousands of unregistered 'care' homes and hospital wards for 'the elderly' where people with dementia languish, and of couples desperately trying to cope with the stark realities of progressive illness, we may be sure that 'projective identification' abounds. However empathetic the 'carer', without support of a psychological, practical and financial kind (in most cases people have difficulty finding money to provide the kind of care that is needed), I doubt they will be constantly empathetic. Kitwood rightly says, referring to 'formal' care, that:

> There can be no question of bolting on a body of knowledge, or of imparting a set of skills in a semi-automated fashion. We are looking for very intelligent and flexible action from a 'reflective practitioner'. The essence of what is required might be described as freedom from ego, so narrow, imperious, conformist, greedy, grasping and demanding. It is under the sway of ego that most people live their ordinary lives. No one is to be blamed for this; it is often a matter of survival, and to some extent it is what being a member of our kind of society involves.
>
> (1997: 131)

Does this sound like the average member of staff, untrained, unsupported and badly paid in the average care home? Kitwood puts his finger on the problem when he points out that being under the sway of 'ego' is often a matter of survival. What better feeding of individual and corporate egos than the obsession with league tables, competition and restriction of resources that blights our health, social and educational services? In an advanced capitalist society, such as Britain, it is inevitable that people deemed 'non-productive' will be 'a big problem', and something has to be done. We don't have workhouses now (or at least they are not so labelled), and it is doubtful whether someone whose perception and co-ordination is very disturbed could be found a useful occupation. It is also the case – see the interviews with Kamal Beeharee (Chapter 11) and Neil McArthur (Chapter 8) – that the idea of having well-trained, well-paid staff for the important job of caring for people with dementia still raises eyebrows. It's not uncommon to find nursing staff with very limited English language in wards with severely dementing people. I came across such an instance recently. When questioned, a manager replied: 'Well they don't understand anything anyway, do they?' And presumably they don't need to be understood. That could apply equally to the patients and to the nurses, neither of whom are being cared for in this situation. I do not wish to put myself on the moral high ground here, claiming any prizes for understanding and empathy, for I have often failed miserably in both. I also make no apology for the often bleak and very negative picture I have presented here. That does not mean that I have subscribed to the 'no hope' culture, because there are indeed patches of light, in the form of better housing and attention to the psychological state of people with dementia (such as provided by Anchor Trust[2]), but these are few and far between. Ten years ago when I had very little knowledge of progressive illnesses such as Parkinson's and Alzheimer's, and of dementia, and indeed didn't want to think about it, I was still horrified at the conditions in 'wards for the elderly', but the full implications of these frightening illnesses only became apparent from close-up involvement. Who would really want to investigate, to get up close, if they didn't have to? Sometimes fate determines that we will become involved, however painful. Let us not pretend that it is easy for anyone, not least the person who is suffering from a progressive illness.

This close-up position is shared by the authors represented in this book, to whom I am very grateful. They have been, and most still are, close to people with progressive illness, often as both personal carer and professional. Nancy Tingey (Chapter 12), whose husband has Parkinson's, has used her experience as an artist and art teacher to establish an art workshop for Parkinson's sufferers in Canberra, Australia. Realising that as well as the important opportunity for involvement in creative processes that the group provided there was a further dimension to the work, she took the opportunity through a Churchill Fellowship to learn about art therapy and committed herself to an intense period of research and personal discovery. The changes she has made to her group define it as an excellent example of 'art as therapy', for Nancy is clear about her boundaries and this makes the group a safe place. Nancy mentions the pioneering work of Ursula Hulme, a founder member of the British Association of Art Therapists, whose association Conquest[3] has, for well over twenty years, quietly and steadily benefited thousands of people suffering the effects of strokes, Parkinson's, multiple sclerosis and other disabling conditions. An artist herself, obliged to flee from the Nazi regime, Ursula has used her creative energy to astonishing effect. Conquest was giving 'care in the community' well before this term was officially coined. Nancy pays tribute to the work of Rita Simon, founder member and Honorary President of the British Association of Art Therapists, who also endured the loss of her husband through Parkinson's. Attilia Cossio from Italy (Chapter 4), another art therapist whose husband suffered from Parkinson's, used her research experience, her knowledge of anthroposophy and her own love of art to set up a project in Milan – and has shared her work generously with ourselves and with others wishing to 'make a difference'. Dorothy Jerrome (Chapter 13), an anthropologist, sociologist and dancer, thought about her own involvement with therapeutic circle dance and worked out how it might benefit people with dementia in terms of movement and social interaction. Starting from a position of 'not knowing' she observed, listened and learned from the participants. Jill Bunce (Chapter 3), trained as a dance movement therapist and became involved in work with Parkinson's as a student. Realising she needed to learn more about her patients' difficulties, she teamed up with neurologists and continues to persevere, bringing a wealth of dance, neurological and movement analysis skills to her groups.

Wendy Magee (Chapter 5), an experienced music therapist, gives us a thorough account of the stages of Huntington's disease, perhaps one of the lesser known progressive illnesses, and shows how music therapy can be helpful in these different stages. John Tyler (Chapter 6) presents an art therapy group. He has worked for more than ten years with elderly people with dementia, noticing the positive effects of art therapy on a range of difficulties. Hearing John talk about his work was a major stimulant for setting up the pilot art therapy research project described in Chapter 10, as despite his careful observations and reports he found it hard to convince other professionals of the value of art therapy. Finlay McInally in Chapter 10 (vignette) and Barry Falk (Chapter 9), co-workers in the new art therapy project, write of their experience in running groups. Both are artists and art therapists, and they bring a careful, sensitive and empathetic approach – just as Kitwood describes as the ideal. Ken Evans, anthropologist, sociologist and psychologist, writes passionately about his ideas and experiences in Chapters 2 and 7, and lets us share his indignation. Ken's front-line experiences and his desire to make sense of them in socio-political terms is well described in his chapters, and he echoes the thoughts of many other authors, including myself, on the 'system failures' in our health and social services. In my own chapters (1, 10 and 14), I have presented thoughts on what it means to have a progressive illness; an art therapy research project in which the team come from very different disciplines: experimental psychology and art therapy (this same team are now involved in a two-year funded project to develop the work of the pilot); and a personal account of living with a partner with progressive illness. I confess that though painful to write, the last chapter had a cathartic effect and I hope it will be of use to other 'carers' who feel themselves less than perfect.

The interviews with Kamal Beeharee (Chapter 11) and Neil McArthur (Chapter 8) are presented in almost exactly the form of our conversations – with some small bits of tidying for clarity, but with questions raised and unanswered as well. I want to thank them both very sincerely for the quiet, persistent and determined attitude they bring to their jobs. They are truly empathetic people, who inspire by their honesty and desire to learn.

This book is limited in its discussion of progressive illnesses mainly to those where dementia is often an outcome. Parkinson's, Alzheimer's and Huntington's diseases are emphasised, while it is acknowledged that other conditions, such as stroke, multiple sclerosis, cancer, severe heart disease, motor neurone disease, involve equal distress for sufferers and their carers. There is a scarcity of literature in the arts therapies on all these conditions and I hope that this will be remedied.

This book is a tentative move towards redressing the balance from those interventions which of necessity deal with the overt physical difficulties and cognitive impairments towards the emotional and philosophical issues which arts therapies are also concerned with. It does not attempt to provide information which can be found elsewhere (such as in-depth medical and biological information on the illnesses discussed and their medication), though individual authors do provide some material which they themselves have found helpful to their own work. Rather, it focuses on the experiences of the authors and their clients and relatives and their struggle with making sense of their worlds.

The book focuses on the 'non-verbal' arts therapies, especially on the role of art, dance, art therapy/psychotherapy, music and dance movement therapy with progressive illness, while recognising that important work is going on in poetry, drama and dramatherapy. The authors are all multi-qualified – I did not realise this until recently when it struck me that we often combine two, three and sometimes four professional or academic disciplines as well as having responsibility for a relative with a progressive illness. I believe that we need to bring together the natural sciences, medicine, social science and the creative arts, not only to treat and care for people with progressive illness but as an antidote to the bureaucratising of our lives – as is well described by Ken Evans in Chapters 2 and 7. There are signs that the medical profession is seeking to broaden its training (for example, a Centre for the Humanities in Medicine has been established at University College London in October 2001), while at the same time having to be deeply cautious of its professional 'image'. Involvement with the arts could, we hope, become a 'normal' aspect of life in the home, in residential care, in hospital, helping to make the lives of those unlucky enough to suffer a progressive illness at least more bearable.

Notes

1 In 1997 the Act of Professions Supplementary to Medicine was extended to include Art, Drama and Music Therapy, and a federal Arts Therapists Board was established under the Council for Professions Supplementary to Medicine. It is a requirement for all arts therapists practising in health, social services and prison services to be state registered. With the passing of the Health Act in 1999, a new Health Professions Council is being established in April 2002, which will replace the CPSM. At that point it is hoped that dance movement therapists will also be able to be regulated.

2 The Anchor Trust has for thirty years provided a range of support, housing and care services to older people throughout England. One of its range of services is Anchor Homes, providing a choice of either residential or nursing care services, with a 24-hour support. Their homes are well designed with modern furniture and facilities, and purpose built for the needs of people with dementia. Many of the homes allow pets, very important for the residents. The aim is to provide a stimulating environment and one in which the quality of life for individual residents is given high priority. Address: Anchor Trust, Chancery House, St Nicholas Way, Sutton, Surrey SM1 1JB, UK.

3 Conquest: The Society for Art for Physically Handicapped People, is a charity which has been providing art classes for both physically handicapped and elderly people for over twenty years. Although not art therapy in its strictest sense, the

groups provide a place for people to release their tensions and frustrations, meet others and counteract the isolation which often accompanies a debilitating illness. Address: Conquest Art Centre, Cox Lane Day Centre, Cox Lane, West Ewell, Surrey KT19 9PL, UK.

References

Bion, W. (1957) Attacks on linking, in *Second Thoughts*. London: Heinemann.

Henzell, J. (1997) Art, madness and anti-psychiatry: a memoir, in K. Killick and J. Schaverien *Art, Psychotherapy and Psychosis*. London: Routledge, pp. 176–197.

Killick, K. (1997) Unintegration and containment in acute psychosis. In K. Killick and J. Schaverien *Art, Psychotherapy and Psychosis*. London: Routledge, pp. 38–51.

Kitwood, T. (1997) *Dementia Reconsidered: The Person comes First*. Buckingham: Open University Press.

Miesen, B.M.L. (1992) Attachment theory and dementia, in G.M.M. Jones and B.M. Miesen (eds) *Caregiving in Dementia*, vol. 1, London: Routledge.

Miesen, B. (1999) *Dementia in Close Up*. London: Routledge.

Resnik, S. (1992) The space of madness, in M. Pines (ed.) *Bion and Group Psychotherapy*. London: Routledge, pp. 220–246.

Schaverien, J. (1997) In K. Killick and J. Schaverien (eds) *Art, Psychotherapy and Psychosis*. London: Routledge, pp. 13–37.

Segal, H. (1975) *Introduction to the Work of Melanie Klein*. The International Psycho-Analytical Library. London: Hogarth Press and the Institute of Psychoanalysis.

Sinason, V. (1992) *Mental Handicap and the Human Condition: New Approaches from the Tavistock*. London: Free Association Books.

Skailes, C. (1997) The forgotten people, in K. Killick and J. Schaverien (eds) *Art, Psychotherapy and Psychosis*. London: Routledge, pp. 198–218.

Terry, R. and Katzman, R. (1992) Alzheimer's disease and cognitive loss, in R. Katzman and J.W. Rowe (eds) *Principles of Geriatric Neurology*. Philadelphia: F.A. Davis and Company.

Wood, C.J. (1997) The history of art therapy and psychosis (1938–95), in K. Killick and J. Schaverien (eds) *Art, Psychotherapy and Psychosis*. London: Routledge, pp. 144–175.

Chapter 2

In the waiting room of the Grim Reaper

Ken Evans

Among the bad habits of sociologists is the tendency to label things in such a way that the complexity of social experience is constrained in discrete and defined boundaries. Some of the consequences of this are that social life is presented (represented) as being much tidier than it actually is, and that social activity and social action is fragmented. Evidence of this tendency can be seen in the titles of sociological studies, claiming to be 'The Sociology' of 'this', 'that' or 'the other'. At present there is no Sociology of Dementia, but when it arrives, no doubt it will conform to the standard format, even down to its title.

The bureaucratic ethos[1] of modern academic sociology has made it a tidy discipline, systematically categorising and filing topics in an orderly way. So when the 'research technicians', aptly identified by C. Wright Mills,[2] finally settle on 'dementia' as a research topic it will probably be filed in a sub-folder under 'Mental Illness', thus isolating it from other social activities. It will then be used by other 'research technicians' to write more books and referred to in government policy documents, but it will not really change anything in the lives of people suffering, directly or indirectly, from dementia.

A reflexive approach would attempt something more general, and attempt to explore rather than examine, and, more importantly, to step over the boundaries that limit our understanding of social activities. It would attempt to locate varied experiences and realities, and identify varied perspectives and explore how these contribute to real-life situations. It would include and compare insiders' views with those from outside the situation. Briefly, it would attempt to reveal the partial and shared views of reality as channelled through one singular concept – that of dementia. Rather than being bound by 'theory' and 'method', it would draw insights from any reference point and incorporate meaning and nuance imaginatively. For what is generally understood as social life is held and expressed in bundles of images, sometimes fleetingly caught, other times slowly burned into our memories and understanding. It is frequently forgotten that images live in the imagination; they are not filed as static reference points, but are active and demanding and compete with all the other images that fill our minds.

From a reflexive approach a sociology of dementia would begin by evoking the most obvious sensation of waiting. Waiting, for whatever purpose, is wasted time. In everyday life waiting for a bus, a train, a plane, at a checkout, a haircut, the dentist, or whatever, means that we are immobilised, unable to do anything purposeful. We accept it passively, but if anything happens to extend our waiting time we complain, sometimes actively and aggressively. Sometimes we use the term loosely to explain a forthcoming event, but in fact we are not really waiting for it, the future event is going to happen anyway, and meanwhile we are getting on with our lives, doing other things. A recurring image I have of dementia sufferers is of their relentless waiting. I have seen it in care homes, hospitals and even in their family homes. Men and women, seated, standing, shuffling from one wall to another, in corridors, dinning rooms, bathrooms, lavatories, sitting rooms, TV rooms, waiting waiting waiting. For dementia suffers all rooms are waiting rooms and all time is waiting time. Each time I visit a place of their suffering, for waiting is part of their suffering, the images are refreshed, and also at other times, when viewing a printed photograph illustrating an article on dementia in a newspaper or magazine, it is always of people waiting. It is at these times when physically removed from a real situation, and having the images refreshed by an externalised image, such as a photograph, that the significance of waiting assumes other meanings.

Would it be too cruel, I wonder, to ask why they are waiting? Sociologists avoid the abrupt question, preferring to speculate on other possibilities. Waiting to eat perhaps, to have a bath, to go to bed, they might suggest. No, not waiting to die, anything but that, and not waiting to connect, to relate to someone, to respond, to think, to be. No, none of these things because a 'what' answer also demands a 'why' answer, and that would be that it is we who make them wait. Perhaps sometimes individually, but always collectively as members of society, a society that imposes the regimen of waiting. The images are too available to permit denial, but uncomfortable images can be shuffled between those with more appeal and, like words, can be used to divert our attention. Making the connection between waiting and suffering might appear to be more psychological than sociological, hence we should begin with some analysis of the basic social unit, the family. Perhaps so, as long as we do not lose sight of the notion that families are in many ways a microcosm of wider society, and that prevailing social values and attitudes, while not necessarily originating in the family, are expressed and made real through the intimacy of family life.

Sociological studies of families are varied, and reflect the whole spectrum of sociological approaches. Although generally they tend to concentrate on structure, depicting families in many modes, it is possible to read between the lines and glimpse something of the varieties of quality of life and relationships.[3] One of the important aspects of families, whatever they are, is that they provide an emotional base-line through which we understand our earliest relationships. It is also through these early relationships that we begin to make sense of ourselves and our wider society. This is what is meant by primary socialisation: becoming a member of a family is the way we become members of society. But initially, of course, we are unable to distinguish the difference between family and wider society. It is only after we have internalised the so-called norms and values of society, as filtered through the perceptions of our parents, that we construct within the family group some idea of who we are – in standard sociological terms a social identity. But in an ideal sociological world norms and values would be less transparent and less pluralist, and the relationship between social values and social action more understandable. Actually sociologists can only guess at this connection.

I find it puzzling to re-read some of the wooden studies of families that I was expected to read as a sociology student. Their mechanical descriptions of conjugal roles, and what brothers and sisters can and cannot do, seem to me almost meaningless now. They rarely referred to how emotional attachments were formed, experienced and changed. Something strange happens when the cold hand of analysis translates human actions into sociological statements. And although I was aware of an ideological underpinning to these studies, I was often encouraged against my own instincts that this was relatively unimportant. My problem now is in making sense of how family ties can become so diminished that more than half of the 600,000 dementia sufferers in this society are abandoned to care homes.

We might wonder if care homes came into existence as a consequence of the diminishing importance of the modern family, or should we somehow blame modernisation for the ways we have become? In functionalist theories the family exists as a sub-system of wider society, and that as society changes so do the functions of the family change. In other words, changes in family life are driven by society. As Parsons, a leading functionalist theorist argues, the isolated nuclear family has been shaped to meet the requirements of the economic system, and is now a small streamlined unit, not encumbered by binding obligations to a wider network of kin. This explanation as least recognises that there are economic pressures shaping social institutions, but his analysis views these modernising forces as positively good for society, and therefore beneficial for families. It also assumes that families are a standardised unit, formed by individuals to serve society.

Whatever the reasons and causes, for example contraception, secularisation, changing work patterns, etc., we all know that the modern family has shrunk. But it is impossible to draw any conclusions about how these changes affect the quality of emotional ties between family members. Certainly in larger families it is possible and desirable economically to care for its members in their home. And to some extent this might explain why the nuclear family, without its extended support facilities, is unable to absorb the extra responsibilities of providing full-time care for someone with dementia. But it does not explain how and why the system and methods, and the quality of residential care, have become the way they are.

From the outside residential care homes often have the appearance of small friendly family hotels. Wherever they are located they seem to belong to the seaside, with its suggestions of fun and relaxation, and something extra, buried deep in the folds of our minds, the association of the seaside and its healing powers. The names carried by these places reinforce the image, sometimes with great subtlety, combining in a single name the benefits of warmth, homeliness and grandeur. Whatever their shape and size they manage to communicate this image of relaxed domesticity. There would be rich pickings for the eager research technicians were they to lift the lids on these places, for these institutions have their own separate history and sociology.

They came into existence in the 1960s in their various forms, their owners converting them from bed-sits to care homes because, with a little effort, they would considerably increase their profit. This was the age of the landlord, a by-product of government policies on homelessness and community care, and residential homes became an extension of the same policy. During this time residential homes sprang up in profusion, and were filled with clients from the DHSS. From the government's viewpoint a simple solution to meeting care and housing needs; from another, a new way of making money. But their rapid growth and reputation was so alarming that the government was forced to introduce measures to 'regulate' their conduct, through the Registered Homes Act 1984, and a publication titled *Home Life*, a recommended code of practice. Again it is necessary to read between the lines of these documents and of local authority policies for residential care, and also the piles of reports of the local Social Services Inspectorate. For between these lines are the clues of personal biographies, of their daily routines, the so-called 'care-plans', the ups and downs of individuals' daily lives, and the dates of their release from the monotony of their existence.

Apart from the few brief handwritten letters of appreciation from residents' families, sometimes pinned to the noticeboards on the entrance walls of some of the homes, there are few written records of how suitable these places might have been. To say that some were better than others is not saying much, because it is impossible to gauge what it is really like to be on the receiving end of their services. The range of perceptions about 'life' within did not include residents' views, but were constructed by those who operate the system – from those who own and run the places, the staff, care managers, inspectors. By the time the system had reached its full machine-like efficiency in the 1980s it was accommodating over a quarter of a million persons, described in government documents as 'the most vulnerable people in our society'. Legislation required homes to be registered, and elaborate procedures were developed by local authority bureaucracies to screen and test and check for non-compliance to regulations. The emphasis was on maintaining the regulations, not on the quality of care, and, like all bureaucracies, in protection from public criticism and legal challenge.

To focus briefly on the relationship between the regulating authority and the homes' owners, which is only one part of the system, is not a deviation; rather, it enables us to come near to the heart of the matter. It seems now that the 1960s had been a watershed for several strands of social change, especially in public opinion and social attitudes – attitudes to love and marriage, divorce, work and leisure, family life, personal relationships. This was also the time when Western national governments ceased to be the driving forces of societies. They continued to perform the administrative functions, but the real influence had shifted to the marketplace, to the large international corporations. For it is they who controlled the media, and called the shots for those who set the trends. This was the time when complete communities were closed down as the investment managers closed mines and factories, and governments were helpless to do anything about it other than maintain law and order. To some ways of thinking it might be difficult in making the connection between the so-called gnomes of Zurich and the plight of an anonymous elderly dementia sufferer, but the link, as Marx would say, is the 'cash-nexus'.[4] Profit, that essential unity that binds everything within the capitalistic system tightly together.

To put it another way, what the elderly dementia sufferer gets in the way of care is what the market permits. Care homes are primarily businesses. Deals are done between local authorities – the purchasers of care and homes, that allows them (the homes) to make some profit. The more problems an individual has (the correct term is 'levels of dependence'), the higher the price. On one side the purchasing authority goes for the maximum 'care' for the minimum price; from the other side the 'providers of care' go for the highest price the market will stand, with the least amount of hassle. When demand for places exceeds availability, the behaviour of competing care managers resembles that of the money-market dealers. Some local authorities purchase 'a block of beds' for a set price, to be filled as the queue of sufferers filters slowly through the system. The shortage of beds, especially those EMI (elderly mentally ill) registered, impinges on registration and inspection issues. Some local authorities cannot afford to close homes, for there is no alternative form of containment. That does not mean that some individuals in the system are not concerned with the quality of care. The phrase is part of their professional language, and certainly some show concern when discussing these issues, but they all work within a system, so real concern becomes one of the pressures of the job. From bottom to top, the system appears to be fulfilling its legal requirements. The Lilliputian individual workers play their individual parts, so when a problem occurs, when something goes wrong, like antibodies they rush to the defence of the system.

Although Social Services care managers have remarkably little direct contact with dementia sufferers, it is through them that placements are made, and they also maintain the formal and informal links between their clients and clients' families. There is no personal involvement because they are functionaries of a system, a bureaucracy, an organisation. Social Services is an institution and deserves a 'sociology' of its own. Weber, one of the founding fathers of sociology, pointed out that the key feature of modern bureaucracies is that they are hierarchical, with specialised roles. These roles are defined in terms of expertise, which depends on specialised education and training, which governs a particular way of operating, the application of impersonal rules and discipline. The care manager as bureaucrat is expected to apply rules (policies) impersonally, and to take no account of the individual with whom they are dealing; care managers are also required to obey the rules and carry out their duties in a disciplined way. In Weber's words:

> The decisive reason for the advance of bureaucratic organisation has always been its purely *technical* superiority over other forms of organisation. The fully developed bureaucratic mechanism compares with other organisations exactly as does the machine with the non-mechanical modes of production. Precision, speed, unambiguity, knowledge of file, continuity, discretion, unity, strict subordination, reduction of friction and of material and personal costs – these are raised to the optimum point in the strictly bureaucratic administration . . .[5]
>
> (1914)

Weber described this as an *ideal type*. In reality the relationships between homes and care managers deviate from this, but always at some cost to the system.

Sometimes care managers are forced to compromise their professional ethic to lubricate the wheels of their business. Within any geographical area (locality) served by Social Services, care managers and managers of residential homes develop particular relationships. They acquire their distinct reputations through interactions with one another. Some care managers are seen as harsh, or strict, others as friendly and helpful. In similar ways, managers of homes are labelled as safe, or careless, and by many other descriptions of approval or otherwise. These views become common knowledge among others in the system.

Residential care homes are also institutions, defined by Erving Goffman as *total institutions*. He noticed a similarity between particular types of institutions, such as military establishments, boarding schools, monasteries, prisons and mental hospitals. Residential homes, especially EMI homes, also share these characteristics: daily activities are timetabled, there is clear resident/ staff division, and a common life controlled in accordance with an overall plan for the benefit of the organisation. From the moment of the sufferer's reception to the moment of their departure every physical activity is controlled and watched by others. But, cruellest of all, Goffman describes the moment of reception as an event, as though passing through a barrier from one world to another, where the individual experiences 'a mortification of the self', the 'death' of their previous identity. Where all of the features that combine to give us identity, our social roles, family membership, self-esteem, are eliminated.

But whereas we can understand this brutalising process in prisons and military bases, because it is based on what Foucault has identified as 'punishment and control',[6] the context of the dementia sufferer is different. And because it is different it is more grotesque, because it is done gently and unconsciously, and regarded by the perpetrators as a kindness. At this point sociological explanations begin to fall apart, we are forced to sift through the images that come to mind, perhaps from Hieronymus Bosch or the concentration camps, or Kafka. Imagine what it is like to wake in the morning after arrival, not in one's own bed, and not metamorphosed as a giant insect, but worse, far worse and infinitely more alarming. To find that the last fragile hold on a diminishing sense of self has slipped away. But Kafka's insights are closer to the truth in his description of 'punishment' in his short story, 'The Penal Settlement'. The Settlement is described as the perfect social unit for its purpose, and its method of correction is a marvellous machine with cogs and wheels, and a bed and a harrow. The prisoner is fastened to the bed, and to the harrow containing hundreds of needles which can be arranged in patterns to make a sentence. As the cogs and wheels slowly turn the condemned person, the harrow writes the sentence into the skin of the victim like a tattoo, over and over again, until the individual is able to understand his sentence from the inside.

I have no way of knowing if this is how the arrival is experienced from the inside; all I know is that increased levels of anguish and distress are evident in their body movements and faces, in their eyes and their voices. I have also sensed the fear at the actual point of realisation that they have been put away. One residential home that I frequently visited was always so stretched by staff shortages that they would ask me to transport a 'patient' to the home, which I did on several occasions. Sometimes I was able to chat to them whilst driving, and in every instance they would ask me where we were going. However limited their insight there was an awareness that they were going somewhere; some protested, others simply repeated the question. With one woman it was relentless, getting louder and louder until eventually she was shouting the single phrase, 'I don't want to go.' But the moment of truth was when we arrived and stopped the car – there was always panic and resistance. A palpable sense of being a stranger, as sensed through the mind of a Peter Slavek[7] or a Hans Castorp,[8] a realisation of hopelessness.

I can replay these scenes in my mind anytime. The last mile or so of the journey, the narrowing country lanes, I turn into the drive of the home, doors open, women dressed as nurses, although they are not nurses, hurry towards the car. Their faces probe the car windows and open the door. Sometimes they need a wheelchair, the few possessions are in a black plastic refuse sack.

If this were all, and the last scene that I could recall, it would be painful enough, but there is a legal requirement for admissions. The necessary paperwork that defines the occasion as 'day one', possessions and medicines are checked, the new recruit is led through small groups of residents and taken into their room. There is a checklist that also includes a line, 'Settle the new resident with a warm beverage.'

Perhaps there could even be a sociology of residents' rooms, but it would be very brief, for the similarity between establishments continues down to the size, decoration, and facilities of the rooms. They resemble miniature film sets of a boudoir, the cheapest possible pastel wallpaper, plastic veneered chipboard furniture, a washbasin, sometimes a toilet, a bed; the whole assembly described in the brochure as 'homely'. Homes policies often make the point that residents' rooms are private spaces, but there is never any sense of real ownership; they are nothing like an ordinary domestic bedroom but more like rooms in cheap boarding houses, with unfriendly smells of disinfectant and urine. In some homes there are 'doubles', where two individuals who have lived most of their lives with another partner, a husband or wife, now find that they are part of another relationship, usually without their agreement. Because the primary consideration is filling beds, the choice of partners is a bureaucratic one, based on whichever combination of residents is least likely to cause problems – usually those least able to complain. It is also assumed that dementia sufferers have negligible personal insight, and are unable to express preferences in such choices. There are many ongoing debates about dementia and dementia care, which includes speculation on personal insight and awareness. My own view is that both awareness and insight are not discrete functions but social processes, as features of relationships rather than attributes. A stimulating physical environment and authentic social relationships will enhance insight and awareness. A mind-numbing room shared with an antagonistic partner must count as a double penalty. My first opportunity to consider questions about dementia sufferers sharing a room occurred one evening when I was called to 'deal' with two very frail women fighting. There were two single beds in the middle of the room, side by side. One occupied by a quietly whimpering white-haired woman, and the other by a wild-looking, but equally frail woman, who was abusive, swearing and pulling the other woman's hair. I was told that the fracas had occurred intermittently for weeks, and the care staff believed that it had been provoked by some disagreement. But this evening was particularly bad, and the abusive woman had managed to pull the other out of her bed by her hair. They clearly did not like each other, but it had not occurred to the manager or the care staff that either had sufficient insight to have and be capable of expressing preferences.

Relationships between dementia sufferers in residential homes are as complex as any others in wider society, but in the unreal world of the dementia care home these become exaggerated and distorted. In other types of total institutions there is at least, to some extent, a self-selecting element; for example, in military institutions soldiers view themselves as sharing common aspirations, and frequently come from similar backgrounds. But dementia sufferers come from the whole range of social and cultural backgrounds, and the effects of social class[9] and occupational differences are retained even at advanced stages of the condition. Accents and habits identify persons and define relationships. In one very small home I visited, with eight residents, the mixture was particularly interesting, from a sociological viewpoint, because of the social class extremes. At one extreme of the social scale there was Harold, an old Etonian who had served in the army and been a director of a large manufacturing company. His accent, vocabulary, and manner were strong reflections of his background. He had managed to retain his self-assurance, but was short tempered, and walked around the home inspecting what he believed to be his personal property. He was patronising towards everyone, including the care staff, whom he frequently dismissed (sacked). He expressed his preferences unashamedly at every opportunity, especially whenever he caught sight of another particular resident (a factory worker) whom he obviously disliked. He would hurl insults, which indicated their social differences. One of the other residents was a timid man from the North, who had been a shipbuilder. He was very quiet and withdrawn, and was always the last to go into the dining room for meals and the last to finish; the staff referred to him as 'the straggler'. For most of the time he drifted from one room to another, hovering and never settling. He hardly spoke to anyone, and his Geordie accent had become a murmur. He was the target of another 'bullying' man, who frequently attacked him, sometimes physically, for not answering his questions.

Accents, clothes and manners, or at least the remnants of them, are the social signals that remain even in total institutions, and these partly account for some kind of a social hierarchy for the residents. For example, they decide who sits where in the lounge, the dining room, and who engages in other social interactions. But hierarchies in care homes have several dimensions; including how staff perceptions of particular residents define and label them, and other layers that exist as a consequence of the informal differences between each of the care staff. Resident and care staff interactions unconsciously combine these variables, and influence who gets attention and who is ignored. In a discussion I had during a training session with care staff about how these differences in relationships affect the quality of care, they initially denied that there were any preferences or 'favourites'. But then they went on to elaborate how some residents were more difficult and 'challenging' than others, and that there were others who were 'gentle' and no trouble at all. They were not aware of any contradictions. Trying to understand how these various perceptions interact within a particular social space and within a particular operating structure is the very stuff of sociology. It should be analysable because of the routines and patterns and orderliness, but each discrete interaction, whether it is between two residents or two members of staff, or between resident and staff, is an engagement that frequently has no pattern. It is disjunctive and fragmented, not part of any whole. It is this particular element that differentiates lived experience in dementia care homes from any other kind of institution.

Staff values and attitudes that concern their own lives are carried into the home, and these influence how they perform their tasks. In most homes care staff work in teams and shifts and consequently develop a kind of camaraderie. The heavy physical nature of the work, combined with the anti-social shift system and the low pay, mostly attracts those whose education and experience restricts opportunities for other types of employment. Training is minimal and usually acquired 'on the job', although some owners of care homes will reluctantly pay for the occasional one-day training session. It is not just the cost of the training that concerns them but the effects of a missing 'pair of hands'. Absenteeism and staff turnover is high, and understaffing is the accepted norm. Although there is a legal requirement to inform the registration authority when staffing levels are below safety requirements, the situation is 'managed', sometimes with agency staff, a further drain on profit, or by coping until the next shift. The standards of care are largely set by the home's manager, which in the case of EMI registered homes is necessarily a registered mental nurse (RMN).

The whole range of tasks – assisting with personal hygiene, dressing, meals, · doctors' and dentists' visits, administration of medication, toileting, escorting, changing clothes, checking on personal safety, facilitating social interactions – should be supervised by the home's manager, but in actuality are so continuous and routinised that they require no supervision. The staff/resident ratio should be better than one-to-eight but is usually worse than one-to-twelve, which means that there is rarely time for staff to sit and chat with residents. All of these things conspire to transform the act of caring into one of guarding and constraining. The early morning routine of washing and dressing and breakfast is hectic. So the respite between meals, late morning and early afternoon is best managed by settling the residents into the lounge, or some other general space, under the control of one or two staff. Meanwhile other staff will be released to change bed linen, or bath residents. It should all happen like clockwork, and for most of the time it does, but as mind-numbing as the routine is it is preferable to the panic when there is an incident, an aggressive outburst or a fall. These impose a further strain on staff; a fall usually means a broken femur, or worse, and involves a trip to the local hospital.

Perhaps it is the manic pace of the staff contrasting sharply with the slow motion of the residents, and the endless and purposeless waiting in such places that induce sensations of unreality and fantasy. With these images in mind I speculate on a non-sociological theme of madness, of different types and degrees – not those defined by psychological categories but those without a name, like the nameless demons of another era, another world-view. What progress have we made, exploring and trying to make sense of these fragmentary interactions, when the outside world meets the interior worlds of banished individuals? Where was the madness? As Laing has shown, madness is not a condition, an illness, but the description of a situation, a social interaction.

But there is always reason in such madness. From an Interactionist perspective[10] we do not experience our environment directly, but always through the ideas that we hold about it. As one of the pioneers of action theories, George Mead argued that individuals give meaning to the world (their world) by defining and interpreting it in certain ways. So the meaning of reality is fundamentally the meaning that we *choose* to give it. But that meaning must to some extent be shared. I recall interviewing a hospital patient, John, in his late sixties, who was recovering from a minor operation but had not been discharged because it was suspected that he was dementing. He had a huge bushy beard and laughing eyes that gave him a friendly appearance. When we first met he greeted me like an old friend, and asked me why I had not been in contact. The remains of his lunch were on the table, and when I asked him if he had enjoyed his meal he complained that he had not eaten for weeks. He wanted to chat and he explained that he was in hospital because 'he had caught one' from the enemy. He made several references to the war, and the 'Hun', but was light-hearted about it and joked about the nurses. It was as if I had walked in on a film set, and become entangled in the action, for he could easily have been playing the part of a wartime hero. On the other hand, these delusions and confabulation could have been symptoms of dementia. He explained also how he had come to grow his beard, describing how he had envied the beard of another patient who had been favoured by the pretty nurses. And that was why he had wanted a beard. Certainly he was confused, but the reasoning was clear.

He was discharged to a residential EMI home, initially for observation, although I did not see him for several weeks. But we did get to know each other during the several months I was visiting the home. On the first occasion he told me that he had settled in and was busy on a project, and might need my help. It turned out that the project was to build a boat capable of sailing around the world. The conversations were always sensible and logical, and the discussions about the selection of materials, and the type of tools required to do the job, made sense. But these were delusions, he seemed unaware that he was surrounded by other residents at various stages of dementia – some very advanced, some of them static and making no sense in their repetitive questions, others continuously wandering or interrupting our conversations. When I asked him who these people were, he simply replied that they lived there. His short-term memory was sufficiently intact to be able to hold a long conversation, and his long-term memory sufficiently intact to be able to refer to previous events; but his sense of reality was different to mine. The care staff told me that he was occasionally incontinent, sometimes avoided having a bath, and also sometimes would wander around on a 'walk-about' for no apparent purpose, but otherwise he was 'co-operative', and quiet and 'gentlemanly'.

One of my visits coincided with a visit from his wife, and I was asked to sit with them and have some tea. His wife, although pleasant mannered, was cold and distant, and kept asking me how advanced her husband's condition was. During the 'tea party' she filled in some of the details of John's illness, and how the forgetfulness had made life difficult; but there were no clues about their feeling for each other, and I was puzzled about this. She had brought some chocolate-ginger cake, which she told me was John's favourite, but when she opened the box John paid no attention. She started to cajole him, and eventually demanded that he eat his 'favourite treat', which he did compliantly. At the end of the chat she asked me if John would be staying in the home, telling me that she had already sold the family home and had moved nearer her sister. She also added that the new arrangements, their separation and John's place in the home 'was for the best'. I agreed with her.

During the next few occasions that I was able to see John there was a noticeable change. His mood was sullen, and he was suspicious when I approached him. The staff who were in the vicinity told me that he had become very incontinent, and had begun 'smearing' his faeces on the walls of his room and making a mess on the carpet. And because of this John had been put on 'Stelazine' and other things to quieten him down. All that I knew of John informed me that this behaviour was contradictory: there had been a life-long habit of cleanliness and interest in his appearance, and he had always been 'jolly'. Now he was a different person.

When I spoke to the manager of the home about this, I had to agree that I was not involved with his care, etc., and despite this I made my point that John's incontinence and 'behaviour' was most likely to be the result of the medication, rather than the other way round. It was also suggested that as I was a consultant psychologist that I was 'pulling rank', which I thought was interestingly revealing, confirming my belief that such institutions are mod-elled on military structures. I did not visit the place for a few months, but when I did the major problem being discussed between the staff, and between the manager and a few senior staff, concerned John's changed behaviour. I was intrigued to hear that a new resident, a 'scatty lady', had formed an attachment with John, and that her behaviour, to some extent, had drawn some of the heat away from him. Apparently the lady was a flirt, and had given John the eye, to which he had responded by engaging her in one of the empty rooms. When they were 'disturbed', they were both naked and making serious progress. I was pleased to hear 'that both sets of clothes had been carefully folded and placed on the chest of drawers'. At least it confirmed my belief that old habits about tidiness are not easily shed. But the 'sexual behaviour', which the manager had informed me about was seen as 'abuse', and therefore had to be prevented.[11]

I saw it differently. What I knew of John's life and relationship with his wife was bleak. Possibly one aspect of his dementia had been shaped by that relationship. He might have been looking for love, or something like it, most of his life, and his 'bout of passion' cheered me with the thought of how enduring the human spirit can be. And in that equally bleak home, which seemed even more now like a gulag of hopelessness, John and his lady had rebelled in the last way open to them. I was able to see John briefly, and pleased to see that he looked considerably better for the experience. This was not the last time I saw or heard about John – apparently considerable staff time was being wasted on keeping him under surveillance. I also later learned that John had been invalided out of his regiment during the last war as a result of a bullet wound in his thigh, and had been decorated for his courage. Whereas the Grim Reaper had failed to get him the first time around, he was now condemned to wait in the waiting room, and denied any privileges for the rest of his sentence.

References and Notes

1 C. Wright Mills (1959) *The Sociological Imagination*, Harmondsworth: Pelican. A brilliant analysis of how social enquiry has become standardised and rationalised in order to serve 'whatever ends its bureaucratic clients may have in view'.

2 C. Wright Mills (1959) *The Sociological Imagination*, Harmondsworth: Pelican. Mills identifies the 'research technicians' as those who have been processed by the American college system and become social researchers, acquiring in the process 'an indifference or a contempt for "social philosophy," . . . And being among the humanistically impoverished, living with reference to values that exclude any arising from a respect for human reason' (p. 117).

3 I'm thinking here mainly of the early Young and Willmott studies in East London, and also the work of Peter Townend (for example, *The Family Life of Old People*, London: Routledge & Kegan Paul, 1957).

4 The cash nexus is a kind of shorthand description for the ways that all human action has been penetrated by the values of the marketplace, from the top to the bottom. Rather than Marx's criticisms of capitalism being 'dead and buried', they are even more relevant in their prophetic vision of the increasing threat of globalisation, with its totalitarian control of the world's financial markets.

5 This quote from Max Weber is taken from The Economy and the Arena of Normative and De Facto Powers, 1914. Quoted in G. Roth and C. Wittich (eds) 1968, *Economy and Society*, Berkeley and Los Angeles: University of California Press, p. 973. Also quoted in J. Fulcher and J. Scott, 1999, *Society*, Oxford University Press, p. 645.

6 *Discipline and Punish*, London: Alan Lane (1975). Foucault's analysis of discipline examines how organisations use discipline to control people's activities through control of the body, surveillance and punishment. Control of the body is achieved by organising time and space to suit the organisation; for example, by controlling the day, which is divided into discrete activities. Surveillance in care homes is extended beyond the genuine requirements of residents' safety, and penetrates private space and time.

7 Peter Slavek is the hero, or neurotic victim, of Arthur Koestler's novel *Arrivals and Departures*. He arrives from nowhere, in the capital of a country called Neutralia, and suffers a mental breakdown. His past life is revealed through the therapy he receives.

8 Hans Castorp, in Thomas Mann's novel *The Magic Mountain*, travels to a sanatorium high in the Swiss Alps to visit his cousin for three weeks, but stays for seven years. His waiting time is spent surviving the rarefied and extra mundane routine of daily life.

9 In psychological terms, a sense of self and social identity includes an understanding of where an individual fits into wider society. Manners and attitudes identify class differences, and dementia sufferers even into the final stages of the illness retain these. Surprisingly, this is a neglected area in research.

10 The Interactionist approach was pioneered by Max Weber, who argued that sociological analysis should not start from social structures but from people's actions. Also the influence of William James and Charles Peirce, both Pragmatists, influenced the direction of sociological thinking of the Chicago School, Cooley, Thomas and Mead.

11 Many homes pay lip service to questions about abuse, without considering bigger ethical questions about wider issues relating to care of elderly vulnerable people. Ethics, however we dress up the term, are basically about how people behave towards other people. The existence of institutional care in its present form is ethically indefensible.

Chapter 3

The living death

Dance movement therapy with Parkinson's patients

Jill Bunce

Parkinson's disease is often described by sufferers as a living death. This description follows many years of physical and psychological hardship and dependence on medication, accompanied by a loss of independence and mobility. The illness involves loss of short-term memory, and in the elderly is accompanied by dementia and disorientation. Increasingly, it is an illness which is associated with a younger age group where it appears to follow a physical or mental trauma. I have in my mind vivid mental pictures of the suffering of a young soldier who, when dancing, suddenly stops, is rooted to the ground and cannot move. Only a few years before he had been on active service. The years in between have seen him pensioned out of the army, trying to adjust to a life where his limbs move unpredictably. His has low self-esteem because of a loss of fitness and libido.

There is the picture of an elderly lady who could run in bright black stilettos under a parachute and who, after a fall, lost her memory and was taken into a nursing home, her family unable to cope with a mother who could not remember them. There was a young patient who hoped for death because she could not face the future of uncertainty. Her wish was granted when an old bronchial problem returned.

These are depressing memories and yet working in a dance movement therapy context, and working psychotherapeutically, the research shows that there are benefits to the patients with Parkinson's disease. I will describe a dance movement therapy group set up in the context of an outpatient's hospital group and the research findings that followed. There is still more to discover and research about this illness which, increasingly, will affect a growing elderly population. There is some evidence to suggest that the illness occurs as a response to trauma. During a seminar for the Parkinson's disease research group 'Spring' in 1999, Susan Greenfield related that it could be a reaction to trauma.

Features of Parkinson's disease

Parkinson's disease results in a reduction of the neurotransmitter dopamine in the basal ganglia, one of the parts of the brain which controls movement. This results in stiffness in the muscles, slowness of movement, difficulty when starting movements, and, in some patients, tremor. This in turn will set up other problems: cognitive impairment, difficulty with skill learning and depression. These factors will interfere with comprehension and motivation. Patients with idiopathic Parkinson's disease at post-mortem have Lewy bodies, round concentric inclusions which are found in the substantia nigra (Marsden, 1994). The term Parkinsonism is used for patients who have similar disabilities, yet may not necessarily have Lewy bodies at post-mortem.

Motor function

Parkinson's disease is a syndrome, evidenced by disturbances in motor function, marked by tremor, bradykinesia (slowness of movement), rigidity and impairment of posture. The most common symptom is a progressive slowing of everyday tasks. Dressing takes longer and patients comment on how they cannot move as before. Patients have difficulties doing fine-movement activities, when these involve alternations of movements – such as writing, which becomes slower and smaller (Marsden, 1994). There is a decrease in spontaneous movement, so that when movement does take place it is slow. As the activity takes place, the slowness is reduced. At the beginning of movement akinesia (loss of movement) is marked and so the patient 'freezes'. Akinesia and bradykinesia lead to a variety of symptoms and signs, which are dependent on the body part. Falls are common and balance is impaired, although gait disturbance and falling are not prominent early symptoms of idiopathic Parkinson's disease.

The patient does not swallow as often and so the saliva collects. This causes distressing dribbling. Eating and swallowing are affected because the jaw muscles function more slowly. Embarrassment therefore causes the patient to eat less. The face appears immobile and expressionless and is referred to as 'mask-like'. The patient cannot move the facial muscles, and normal emotions are felt but not expressed. The facial expression can give an impression of dullness, anger or a fixed stare which causes communication problems. Partners seem to be affected by this, in that their reaction to the patient's facial expression is altered. Normal facial movements in social interchange are decreased, or social interchange is limited with partners, relatives and friends because of difficulty in expressing emotion.

The posture and gait of the person can be abnormal. In some, the position is hunched and kyphotic. The hands are held in front of the body and the head bowed. The patient will sit immobile, and getting out of a chair is slow and difficult. In Parkinson's disease, the ability to co-ordinate the initiation of these movements is impaired. Turning over in bed is difficult. There is an absence of spontaneous movement and stiffness is evident, leading to difficulty in finding comfortable positions. The initiation of walking is hesitant, especially in crowds. If walking can be begun, it is impaired after three or more steps. Loss of swinging of the arms whilst walking is one of the earliest signs. Cessation of walking is also difficult; particularly if it is attempted suddenly. The patient cannot adjust the centre of gravity of the trunk in relation to the legs, and this often leads to falls. There is no resistance to being pushed over, as the righting reflex is altered. In about 70 per cent of patients there is resting tremor; which may not reduce with activity. It can cause spills when holding hot drinks in cups and is socially disabling. Rigidity can be a factor in balance ability. The rigidity is caused by an alteration in the descending extra pyramidal motor pathways in the brain. It is not a spasticity. The hypotonia is the same throughout the range of movement.

With progressive disease there is an 'on–off' phenomenon, which is the name given to a sudden improvement and deterioration in bradykinesia. Freezing occurs suddenly and there may not be a quick recovery. Medication may be one of the reasons for the motor fluctuations and is often a feature of patients who have had Parkinson's disease for some time (Quinn, 1990).

Parkinson's disease can be socially isolating: speech can become very quiet and indistinct as rigidity affects the muscles of speech. This in turn causes relatives and partners to feel isolated, and family life can become difficult.

Falling is a multifactorial problem for the Parkinson's patient. Falling causes fractures, which limit mobility and therefore quality of life, which leads to isolation and depression. Although abnormalities of gait and loss of postural reflexes are serious disabilities late in the course of Parkinsonism, they are not obvious at the onset of symptoms. In the early stages, gait and postural reflexes are normal. There might be a slight dragging of one leg or one foot. The early abnormalities are a decrease in arm swing and mild flexion posturing of one arm. As the disease advances, the torso adopts a flexed posture, the stride shortens and the foot slides instead of being lifted. Patients walk on their toes and take short, hurried steps. Turning becomes difficult and the body rotates as a whole instead of the head leading. It takes a few steps to accomplish a turn. If the space is small and confined, a patient's gait deteriorates. Risk factors occur in the environment, such as surfaces, furniture and crowded kitchens.

If the patient has dementia, hypertension, visual and proprioceptive malfunction and musculoskeletal disorders, the problems will be much worse. Poor judgement and inattention contribute to falls. Shuffling and freezing also exacerbate the problem. Freezing may be resistant to pharmacological treatment. Observation of standing and postural reflexes, gait and history of the falls contributes to an understanding of the lack of balance in each patient. Emotional states also seem to contribute towards an inclination to fall (Gancher et al., 1992).

Not only are there physical manifestations of the 'living death' symptoms of an illness, there are also symptoms of depression, catatonia and hysteria. These psychological features of the disease led Charcot to call the illness 'a neurosis' (Charcot, 1880).

The psychological features of the illness are not often addressed, and there seems to be a psychological link to the physical symptoms. The interrelationship between physical and psychological symptoms is generally denied in favour of a focus on the physical. The psychological symptoms of Parkinson's disease are caused by a deficiency of neurotransmitters in the brain.

Some patients do not respond well to drug treatment, and some of their psychological symptoms such as depression and withdrawal seem to influence the effectiveness of drugs. This can be seen in the blunting of drive and lack of response to the outside world, caused by the psychological state rather than by ineffective medication therapy.

It is suggested that other neurotransmitter deficits may be responsible for depression (Marsden, 1994). The fluctuation in levels of serotonin and noradrenaline can cause depression in patients with Parkinson's. Lees and Smith's study (cited in Marsden, 1994), and results of neurological testing, has shown that the psychological features of the illness suggest frontal lobe dysfunction. In the early stages there appears to be little obvious cognitive disability. However, what does develop is a growing apathy (abulia), slowness of thought, and the blunting of drive and response to the outside world. This can increase to an impairment of memory and developing dementia. This curious mix of psychological and motor features has to be taken into account in clinical work, as motor symptoms can indicate psychological disturbance which can affect motor performance.

Movement in Parkinson's disease

The first movement abnormalities to be described were: (a) 'festination', (b) 'pulsion' (Sacks, 1991).

Festination is seen in walking, talking and thinking. Movements are accelerated and abbreviated and give an impression of impatience and urgency, although some patients complain that they are going more quickly than they want. There is also the restlessness, which means patients will change position continually in a chair or be forced to walk around. This is known as akathesia.

In contrast to this are the slowing down of movement and the difficulty in initiating movement. Movement and speech are slowed and the patient freezes and cannot move, complaining of being stuck. Following his own observations, Charcot concluded that the rigidity and akinesia were the outcome of an inner struggle. This inner tension is followed by extreme tiredness. The akinesia causes exhaustion and results from a sense of agitation and alarm (Parkinson, [1817] 1992). Parkinson noticed that patients had little power to move even though motivated. As the debility increases and the motivation fades, the tremor becomes more violent and exhaustion follows. There is a need for a release in sleep. There are sleep disturbances resulting in the patient having little sleep or little relaxation.

Sacks (1991) suggests ways of achieving an understanding of what it is like to be a sufferer. He feels that we must come down from our position as 'objective observers' and meet our patients face to face. He says that we should meet them in a sympathetic and imaginative encounter. He feels that to reach patients the use of images, analogies and metaphors will assist 'to make the strange familiar, and to bring into the thinkable the previously unthinkable' (Sacks, 1991: 3–11).

The movements convey characteristics of resistance, continual repetition and sometimes lack of motion. Patients can sit, appearing apathetic and with no will to move. Sometimes they will move only if someone engages them or orders them to move. There is a dullness of facial expression, lack of energy and an overall feeling of tiredness. There is a lack of expression of emotion, focus and attention. These characteristics are features of the changes caused by the Parkinsonism. There is an alteration in the initiation of movement and a loss of vitality, marked by an absence of impulse in the movement phasing. There is also absence of swing in the arms while walking.

There is a presentation in the pathology of opposites, 'a pathological absence and a pathological presence' (Sacks, 1991: 3–11). This can be seen in a type of 'up and down' behaviour, a swing from an aroused and excited state to one of profound exhaustion and apathy and an almost catatonic state. Extreme passivity is evident. There is a poverty of expression, but movements become over-organised. If patients become involved in a movement process the motor symptoms can disappear for a short time, or the disabilities can lessen.

If involvement alters then the symptoms return. Sacks describes this process as 'an intense pressure that might be relieved or an intense change discharged' (1991: 3–11). These concepts were emphasised by Charcot (1880), who compared the 'phases' of Parkinson's disease with those of neurosis. He named the phases as the compliant-preservative, the obstructive-resistive and the explosive-precipitate phases with the plastic, rigid and frenzied forms of catatonia and hysteria.

There are several reports that there are abnormal personality features such as apathy and depression which antecede the onset of Parkinson's disease, as seen in Lees' and Todes' study (cited in Joseph and Young, 1992), but research has not been able to confirm a pre-morbid personality. If there is, then it takes a long time for the obvious symptoms and motor disabilities to be evident.

Psychiatric features of Parkinson's disease

The psychiatric features of Parkinsonism include depression, psychosis and dementia. The exact frequency of depression is uncertain, although Marsden (1994) says that two-thirds of patients are depressed. Depression is not always due to diagnosis or disability, sometimes it is due to fluctuating levels of neurotransmitters. It has been suggested that death of dopamine cells is not solely responsible for those features, but other neurotransmitters such as serotonin and noradrenaline are affected.

There are a number of neuro-psychiatric problems. Most patients have slight changes on neuro-psychological testing, which indicates frontal lobe dysfunction. There does not appear to be cognitive malfunction early on, but, with time, patients become apathetic, slow in thought and do not react to the environment. According to Marsden (1994), 20–30 per cent of patients may go on to develop dementia. The elderly patient often suffers from confusion.

There are many reasons for cognitive impairment. Some frontal lobe dysfunction may be due to dopaminergic loss. It does appear from recent evidence that Lewy body pathology is more widespread than was thought previously (Marsden, 1994). In those patients with cognitive disability there are widespread Lewy bodies in the cortex. Diffuse cortical Lewy body disease is now thought to be a common cause of dementia in the elderly Parkinson's disease patient.

There are also psychotic symptoms associated with Parkinson's disease, usually in the elderly. Visual hallucinations are common. Patients 'see' figures or people which they might find threatening. These can occur in the day as well as in the night. There are also instances of 'continuous dreams', which can also appear in the daytime. Patients may become psychotic. These symptoms may be due to an excess of drug intake, but these psychotic features are also part of the disease itself.

Anxiety may feature large in the mood changes, especially during 'off' periods. Fear of the unknown and changes within the disease cause anxiety. This anxiety is transferred to other family members, which causes stress and strained relationships. The behavioural changes and the mood swings upset family relationships.

Posture and the therapeutic process

Postural changes in Parkinson's disease can lead to a lack of balance. This lack of physical balance becomes a metaphor for the person's feeling state. Body images provide metaphors which express underlying feelings. The dance movement therapist can address the interrelationship between the motor symptoms and the psychological state when working in the areas of the body structure, movement analysis and the creative process. The creative process uses the body relationships and the psychotherapeutic dynamics underlying the group relationships.

Posture and communication

Parkinson's disease has major effects on posture. The changes in posture lead to a lack of stability and poor communication (Bull, 1987). Changes in posture play a large part in communication and conversation. In conversation and social interaction unconscious movements reflect feelings and responses. Postural changes give messages to other people. Verbal communication is unconsciously influenced by postural changes in others. The disease progression leads to sideways lean. The chin may be slumped forward on to the sternum. There may be an inability to stay upright. Relatives and friends receive mixed messages and communication errors occur. Leaning over sideways may be interpreted as apathy, depression or a feeling of hopelessness. Conversely, patients can have these feelings, and carers may overlook their needs because the positioning is interpreted as part of the disease. Close relatives take on abnormal postures themselves, or become depressed because of the situation and adopt bizarre postures. Bull (1987) has shown the emotional and interactional significance of posture. He found that the role of posture in non-verbal communication has been underestimated. His results showed that both movements and positions convey information about distinctive emotions and attitudes. He demonstrated that posture is a source of information about listener emotions and attitude.

The therapist can use these ideas to elicit response and to aid communication. The therapist's response must include an awareness of her own body's postural shifts and how they can affect communication and mood. The therapist may have to create body postures to assist communication or to elicit response. Posture reflects the severity of the disease. Patients can be made sufficiently aware so that they will make postural adjustments. Even at late stages, posture might be altered by mood, particularly depression. It is important for the therapist to separate both posture and mood to make appropriate interventions. Anxiety can be controlled by breathing techniques. These help to expand the chest, and release tension. Breathing influences body shaping, which in turn relates to mobility and stability. It also emphasises an awareness of weight in the body and can bring an awareness of a shift in weight and how that is utilised and mobilised in the body.

The body is central to an understanding of self and is the central component for movement. The structure of the body influences how we move. If Parkinson's disease patients become aware of body changes they can intervene and understand the process, enabling them to feel that they have more control and consequently lessen their anxiety.

'Our bodies are the reflections of our lives, sitting, walking, standing, we absorb the impact of each day. Each thought and sensation makes changes in the body' (Crickmay and Tufnell, 1990). It has been observed that the use of body images in visualisation also creates a way of loosening the body and mind from the habits of a progressive disease. Body metaphors can be used to create a greater sense of self and awareness of others. For example: 'Standing on my own feet' means I am capable of being independent. 'You are a pain in the neck' means being unable to tolerate another group member. 'I am always falling over' means that I am constantly feeling insecure and live with fear and anxiety. 'I feel I am shrinking' means I am withdrawing from human contact and becoming less important or losing my identity. The body can be a source of imaginative ideas which can lead to a different understanding of being and relating, but also a sound knowledge of the physiology of the body is essential to any study related to the use of the body (Bartenieff, 1980).

In order to engage the body fully it is necessary to use the floor, as some patients experience problems with balance, lack confidence and have a fear of falling. Emphasis is placed on overall mobility. Rather than strengthening selected muscle groups, the body is mobilised as a whole. Muscle groups work together to support movement. Every movement in the body involves movement somewhere else in the body. It is important for the Parkinson's disease patient to become aware of where the movement begins. The patient must be clear about where the movement is going in space. Starting with work on the floor, the patient progresses from floor to standing.

Work on the floor is also important for Parkinson's disease patients because it reduces the need to struggle in order to remain upright. For many patients being upright is an internal struggle which they find exhausting. Floor work reduces the exhaustion caused by the need to participate in everyday life (Bartenieff, 1980). Each of the fundamentals focuses on the overall co-ordination of the body, which again is important for the Parkinson's disease patient. The author has observed that whole body movements give a sense of connectedness in the body and assist the link between the sense of self and body experience. The connectedness in the body allows the 'flow' to complete activation without too much exertion or stress (Bartenieff, 1980).

It is important to note body parts, the movement possibilities of upper and lower body and the movement of limbs. It is necessary to make the patients aware of structures in the body to create more self-awareness. This can be done in a creative way using pictures, photographs and visualisation. These provide a source for improvisation and body contact (Crickmay and Tufnell, 1990).

The work of Bonnie Bainbridge Cohen (1993) explores the relationship between body structure, movement, cognition and emotional response. Her work has its roots in psychological, physiological and developmental principles. It is possible to express feelings and thought through the body. The key concept of dance movement therapy is that there is a relationship between motion, emotion and cognition. Exploring movement in a way which extends a patient's range of movement can assist in an expression of emotion. The patient's feelings can be shared in a symbolic way where words fail and verbal communication is not possible. The body and its structure can be used as a means of symbolic expression. The use of touch can be used in repatterning and extending movement patterns. It was observed by the author that some patients need to re-experience early developmental movements which re-establish early bonding. Through touch, the patient relearns the meaning of tactile experience and how this relates to contact with other people and their intimate relationships. The importance of the skin is described by Montagu (1971). The skin is an organ which is involved in the physical and psychological development of a human being. The lack of tactile experience in infancy can affect the psychological and physical development of the adult (Montagu, 1971).

The brain receives sensory information from the skin, muscles and joints. It then organises these sensations so that a person can move, learn and behave normally. A Parkinson's disease patient's sensory organisation is affected. Sensory information from the skin, muscles and joints is disorganised. This can lead to inadequate perceptions and an alteration in the way the patient relates to people. The skin has a vital role in emotional relationships and the development of feeling secure. Through the skin the patient can relearn how to be intimate and how to make appropriate contact with the environment and other people.

Poor sensory integration affects proper initiation and sequencing, but through the use of developmental work and the stimulation of the senses it is possible to extend a patient's range of movement.

Developmental movement

Some early movement developmental patterns need to be re-experienced in Parkinson's disease patients as there are indications that some stages have been omitted, or need to be reworked. Failing to complete a developmental stage can lead to problems in balance, perception, sequencing, organisation, memory and creativity (Ayres, 1991). These symptoms occur in patients with Parkinson's disease, and developmental work has been observed to assist in extending movement range. Bonnie Bainbridge Cohen (1993) established developmental patterns of movement which correspond to perception and which assist with spatial orientation. Work now being researched by Schore (1994) suggests that the growing brain and attachment patterns in childhood are linked. There is evidence to suggest that the genetic systems that programme brain development are influenced by the post-natal environment. It may be that the development and progression of the illness is connected to early brain development, which relies on early affect relationships. Maturation of an adaptive cortical system is organised and is dependent on early experience and socialisation. It is the social environment that induces the reorganisation of brain structures. The underlying principle of development is, according to Scott (cited in Schore, 1994: 233), that 'there is no reorganisation without disorganisation'. It is possible that the process in the development of the brain is the same process in its degeneration and that its early organisation is responsible for its later disorganisation. The brain is programmed to be sensitive to emotional states and this involves a reorganisation of the circuits of the orbital frontal areas of the cerebral cortex.

During thirty years of research, Kestenberg has linked particular psychological developmental stages to movement. She found that inappropriate movement patterns could delay development or encourage the early formation of rigid defences. In both cases they could encourage fixed personality traits. Children who could not recover from early interference could develop borderline personality disorders or inappropriate defences as adults. Parkinson's disease patients seem to suffer from inappropriate defences and the lack of awareness of the need for boundaries, which could relate to early developmental interference. Kestenberg's work assists the therapist in assessing the patient's needs as well as indicating the developmental stage the patient needs to re-experience (Kestenberg, 1975). The developmental stages are identified through the therapy sessions and assist in the planning of treatment (Loman, 1990).

The importance of emotional stimulus and social interaction is vitally important in the use of movement in the dance movement therapy process. The Parkinson's disease patient is in a similar position to the neurotic patient. The painful contracted muscles become an 'armour' which causes an inability to express emotion and results in a disinterest in the environment and towards people. However, the repeated discharging of emotion, or the physical release of muscles, is not enough. The 'armour' is only relieved temporarily until the underlying cause of depression has been found. It is the role of the dance movement therapist to connect the body experience with the emotional experience and to rework past emotional traumas.

In order to alleviate the depression it is important for the patient to feel safe and secure. The therapist spends time in establishing a good relationship. This assists the patient in dropping their resistance to change and developing trust, so that feelings may be expressed.

The secure environment provides an environment which facilitates the recovery from past traumatic experience. The patient will only be able to do this when inappropriate defences have been removed and appropriate behaviour patterns established. This is assisted by the psychotherapeutic process dynamics of the group. The creative process within the group enables patients to rework their past experiences and find new ways of relating, expressed in movement.

Movement analysis

The therapeutic interventions involved in the movement process are based on Laban's movement analysis and the psychotherapeutic process. It is important to use his ideas because cognitive, emotional and physical states are affected in Parkinson's disease. Laban's analysis depends on how emotional states are reflected in movement patterns. Parkinson's disease patients need to consider the relationship of bodily action and spatial patterns. In Laban's theory there is a correspondence between the mover's use of space and the dynamics in their movements. This concept became the basis of Warren Lamb's work in America (Lamb, 1965). The dynamics of movement are related to the intensity or degree of lability. The four elements of intensity are weight (force), time, space (how direction is used) and flow (flux, lability). These four elements are called 'efforts' (Laban and Lawrence, 1974). The term 'effort' is derived from a concept of striving. Laban analysed these in a system of 'effort' action. In every movement all factors of motion, space, weight, time and flow are present and interdependent (Laban, 1960). The study of elements or 'efforts' is necessary for work with Parkinson's disease because it indicates the types of movements to be used, depending on observation of the patients.

These combined elements can be examined individually or looked at as a combination of dynamics. Together they reflect the patient's inner state. Imbalances occur in body, personality and cognitive ability. This analysis is valuable, for the movement tells us so much about the state of the person in body, mind and feeling. Interventions can then be made according to how the person is using the elements of space, weight, time and flow. This analysis also indicates how the changes in the body can be understood. It may go on to indicate how movement can be used to enable some greater mobility.

The body and its movements become a means of expression, revealing unconscious relationships which communicate where words cannot be used (North, 1972). This is possible in a population which may seem so lacking in expectation as Parkinson's disease patients. The emphasis on an attitude to the environment can direct the movement. This relates to the cognitive capacities of orientating, attending and focusing. The mastery of the environment can give clarity to a patient's alignment and their relationship to the environment. It has been observed that emphasising the spatial element helps a patient's orientation.

An emphasis on weight in the body, where the patient experiences the sense of gravity, helps the patient with stability and sense of balance. Using time qualities indicates a readiness for decision. Parkinson's disease patients have problems with awareness of time and decision-making. Emphasis on flow is associated with feelings which can bring out interactions of self and others. This can lead into more controlled or less controlled movements. Some

Parkinson's disease patients find a freer flow or less controlled movements more difficult. This can cause anxiety or exacerbate the tremor.

Free flow is only used when patients can tolerate losing control, or need to overcome problems with over-control or where the anxiety level is not high. In helping Parkinson's disease patients with emotional problems stability and healthy defence mechanisms have to be secured. Too much anxiety can increase tremor, and a loss of control can cause an increase in physical symptoms depending on the individual. The movements also express the nature and progression of Parkinson's disease. Observation can illustrate the person's movement repertoire. Through experience it has been possible to rebuild the movement patterns. In the movement we can build a picture of the patient's personality before it was 'possessed' by Parkinson's disease, for small movements can still reveal something of the person (North, 1972).

The dance movement therapy process

The Parkinson's condition is synonymous with change because of its progressive nature. In the dance movement therapeutic process, the body becomes a metaphor for the painful feelings caused by the progression of the illness. Body changes caused by the disease can be used as a primary instrument in the therapy. These changes provide metaphors which can be used verbally to reach the underlying feelings which are not expressed. The use of metaphor and imagery in describing movement helps to create a new awareness of feelings. The creation of a new body image comes from an integration of sensation from the outside to the internal world of feelings and experience. Todd, in *The Thinking Body* (1937: 295), states that bodily attitudes affect thinking and feeling: 'Imagination itself, of the inner image, is a form of physical expression and the motor response is the reflection of it.'

Winnicott (1953) traced the relationship between the inner and outer experience to the 'integrating tendencies'. The 'integrating tendencies' are the abilities of people to make sense of overwhelming experiences. The ability to understand and give a structure to their inner world enables them to make changes in their behaviour. These 'integrating tendencies' help the inner world of feeling, and the outer world of experience can be related to one another. Dance movement therapy provides the means of integrating inner and outer experience through movement. A deeper awareness of the body and the awakening of the realisation that there is some control over the illness develops a more positive sense of well-being. The therapist's body becomes a mirror for the patient's movements and a way of experiencing the body experience of the patient. The mirroring reflects back to the individual, in the group, the emotional content of the session. The movements act as a container for the expression of difficult feelings, such as a loss and fear, and facilitate the development of a psychodynamic process. The symbolic meaning of the metaphor expressed in the movement is made sense of in the verbal process and is interpreted by the therapist. The interpretation is reflected back to the patient through movement, which has metaphoric value and can be verbalised either by group members or therapists. This process extends the group members' movement repertoire and accesses emotions: it is creative because it incorporates new ideas, awareness of feelings and the way they are expressed.

Clinical context

The research is based on work at a Midlands hospital, 1992–1996, private practice from 1992 until the present day, and during three therapeutic holidays for Parkinson's disease patients, 1998, 1999 and 2000. The clients are both young-onset and elderly. The holidays provided a variety of approaches such as art therapy, performance skills, sport and outdoor pursuits, and speech therapy as well as dance movement therapy, folk and social dancing. In addition there was massage and gentle exercise classes. There was group, individual and marital therapy. People attended for short- or long-term work, depending on their needs and suggestions from the neurologists. There has been some input from the Parkinson's Disease Society in recommendations of clients for the holidays. The holidays were a week long and were for patients, carers and their families. Some of the work was in a family context, some in separate groups for patients and for relatives. There was a considerable amount of work done with the children, who were with single parents and who were the carers of young-onset patients.

The structure of a group session

1   warm up;
2   movement process;
3   verbal closure.

The warm up is particularly important and careful attention has to be made to the anatomy of the body, with careful preparation in order to warm up the muscles and to be gentle with joints that are difficult to move. The type of movement introduced is important, as movement can assist in mental associations. This can be seen when strong direct movements can elicit feelings of frustration and anger. The movement process began with the use of balls, parachutes, elastic and stretch cloths. The use of balls seems to be useful as it has been observed that fast-moving objects engage the patients. This is probably due to the 'paradoxical movement' whereby patients can suddenly run if there is a fire or an emergency. The use of improvised play with balls provides a visual focus in the session. This seems to engage them emotionally. The use of the parachute, elastic and stretch cloths brought the group together and helped patients to work together. This part of the session allowed people to play, which stimulated fantasy and creativity within the group. Play provided experience for the use of metaphors, descriptions and stories in the verbal process. This kind of experience was used in the verbal process to gain insight and to bring areas of conflict into consciousness. The play integrated the cognitive, emotional and behavioural aspects of the patient.

In the verbal process many clients had difficulty with speech: the voice can be so quiet that no one can hear. It is difficult to move the tongue and lips, causing problems with articulation. Some patients suffering from dementia found it difficult to express themselves. However, the value of stories and reviving past memories was crucial to these clients (Hodgkinson, 1994). Movements can motivate patients into expressing themselves. The opportunity to have an active part in creating stories, particularly from the patient's past, assists in making the patient feel better and puts them in touch with their feelings. Acting out through movement can provide rich emotional experience, which can be processed in the verbal part of the session. The verbal process should not be considered as separate from the movement but as a development from it. It helps to clarify and explore what happened during the movement. The metaphors from the movement provide rich emotional material which can be used to address personal and group issues. The verbal process gives insight to the group dynamics and an opportunity for the individual to understand their own emotions so that over a period of time the clients become more self-aware.

It was important to keep to time boundaries and to keep to the same room space. The disease gives to patient and carer a feeling of being out of time; not belonging to life. They seem to have no sense of time. From the work on space and time boundaries, the group members experienced constancy, which assisted in a sense of security. This gave a feeling of a safe space where feelings could be explored. At first, patients resented the emphasis on time boundaries and carers would often try to go on talking when the sessions had finished. The resentment passed and patients began to like the sense of order. In the discussion that followed the movement, the clients related the body to 'body metaphors' – for example, 'standing on my own feet' (meaning 'I have a need to be independent'). Many patients had lost touch with themselves or did not relate to their misshapen bodies. One of them said, 'I feel like a shrinking violet' and related that to a withdrawn state. There was time for long-term clients to reintegrate emotional traumas that seem to proceed their illness. There seemed to be many clients with unresolved, multiple losses.

Case study

M. is 63 years old and has had Parkinson's disease for sixteen years. She came to my group at the hospital in 1992. Her walking was stiff and slow, her hands had stiff joints. She would hide them or cover them up. She complained about feeling cold and she would spend most of the time hidden away at home, covered in layers of clothes, still feeling the cold. When I first met her she seemed depressed, withdrawn, hardly speaking and her facial expressions spoke of anxiety. She suffered from claustrophobia and still does. She had problems with balance, tripping and holding objects. She had rarely attended the hospital in eight years because of a lack of clinic facilities, and her drug programme had been not been monitored regularly. She had begun to attend the new consultant's clinic in October 1992, and since then she has had changes to her medication. She was found to be suffering from low blood pressure. She has continued to attend regular clinics and in 1998 she ceased coming to my group because she wanted to look after her grandchild. She left the group, with regrets, but with a hope for the future. She still acts as a babysitter and, despite problems with walking and a few complications with drugs, continues to have an active life. She was recommended to attend the outpatient dance movement therapy group by her consultant in 1992. This referral was part of the institution of a new policy by the consultant who wanted to use therapies alongside a drug programme. The aim of this initiative was to reduce the amount of prescribed drugs.

Family history

She was born in a northern manufacturing town. She was an only child. Her father died a few years ago of leukaemia, and her mother died three years ago. She is happily married and her husband retired to help her with the Parkinson's disease. She has one adopted son, who is in his early thirties, married with one child, and is a policeman. When her mother died she experienced some emotional relief, as their relationship was stormy, and in M.'s early life her mother had been abusive. M. described the moment when she could feel the sting of her mother's wedding ring on her face, when she had been slapped as a child. When her mother had come to stay her Parkinsonian symptoms worsened.

M. had a stillbirth at her home, and her mother's response had been to shut the door and let her 'get on with it' without seeking medical advice. As a young child, M. was tied to a bed. This memory seems to have been the trigger for her claustrophobia. Her relationship with her adopted son is good and she enjoys the new hope that her grandchild has brought. She has moved house several times because of her husband's job. Moving house seems to be a common trigger for the development of the illness. According to her, the illness began when she moved to Oldham. She describes it as a cold, isolated and polluted place. It became a symbol of her feelings of coldness and rejection.

Treatment

She attended the dance movement therapy group once a week. When she first attended her movements were minimal, ill-defined, very slow and unsure. Her movements were gestural and peripheral to the body. The movements in the top half of the body were not co-ordinated with the ones at the bottom. She dragged one foot, but eventually she learned to cope with this and it did not prevent her from being active. She did have a propensity to fall. She did not use the centre of her body at all; this indicated some deep emotional problem. It was as the therapy continued that I learned of her abuse and the problems that she was having with her mother. It was after a bad attack of enteritis that followed a stressful time with her mother that she was diagnosed with Parkinson's disease.

Clinical progress

She has worked through her feelings of bereavement, working on the losses of her father and mother-in-law. She has worked on other feelings of loss: loss of youth, loss of her abilities, and loss of employment. She has been able to work through these feelings in a safe and supportive environment. She complains less about the attacks of enteritis, and seems more able to deal with stress, particularly in personal relationships. She has become a support to others and gives talks to local support groups. She is no longer withdrawn or depressed and has become outgoing. She has developed some mastery and control. Her movements have become graceful and she is now able to use her hands, knitting garments and making hats for a wedding. Her movements are more co-ordinated, and she likes to touch and experience different materials. I feel, even though she asked to leave the group to look after her grandchild, she showed a sense of direction and purpose. She left with a greater sense of self-esteem and well-being.

Discussion

The group, individual and family work offered hope when the condition seemed hopeless. The dance movement therapy process revealed to the therapist issues of the patient, carer and family which seemed to influence motor abilities and the ability to cope with this insidious, progressive illness. Research and therapy work which has been completed in the last eight years has shown that the issues that influence disease progression are:

- The need for a positive outlook in coping with the disease.
- The need for support.
- The need for communication and socialisation which enabled them to develop their emotional life, which in turn seems to stimulate brain activity.

- The need to alleviate depression and withdrawal which prevents stimulation and maintaining an active life.
- The need for clear boundaries in order to create a safe environment to alleviate stress caused by past traumas.
- The reworking of defence mechanisms so that inappropriate defences could be removed and more appropriate ways of coping established. A better management of the illness seems to be crucial to the progression. The patient needs to be able to feel they are in control and have active participation in decisions about their own lives. The feelings of embarrassment, self-consciousness, loss and bereavement need to be explored. These feelings can be as disabling as the motor problems.
- Restrictive family patterns which encouraged dependency or a lack of self-motivation need to be deconstructed, but sensitively and slowly enough so that there is no sense of attack or increase in anxiety. This was achieved by the patients and carers reworking past family relationships. Dysfunctional patterns were reshaped, patients and carers were able to cope more easily with the disease.

The groups

The therapist's work was client centred. The patients who had suffered abuse or psychological rejection benefited from this positive regard. Standal (1954) defined 'positive regard' as the need to feel worth about ourselves, which comes from significant others in childhood. Alongside the need for positive regard, there develops the need for self-regard. Patients need to feel good about themselves despite a debilitating illness. If this need is not met, it becomes difficult to function in the environment because of a lack of confidence. Those patients who received only selective positive regard in childhood found it difficult to maintain self-regard. The patient, who is surrounded by criticism and disapproval by confusing and ambiguous messages from the carer, becomes confused. The carer who is over self-critical and lacks self-worth will find caring a burden. Both will be anxious and trying to attract ways of discovering attention or signs of discovering affection. The positive regard from the therapist may be the first time that the patient is given value. Patient and carer become less self-punishing and lose the guilty sense that the illness was a punishment for their 'sins' and past actions. Parkinson's disease patients often lack motivation because they feel that there is no longer any point to their lives and that the future is bleak because of a progressive disease. When they become more active and can maintain functional abilities they then can develop a sense of hope which enables them to take part in life. The groups which were researched developed a sense of sociability and began to visit theatres and take part in fund-raising events. Several clients have established support groups which have continued with their participation. These groups now raise money for research and because they have learned about group dynamics within the therapy groups by being an active member of a group they have become empowered to work together to help each other.

The method of evaluation was empowering, as interviews and questionnaires were used as a means of evaluation. The evaluation showed that there had been improvements in motor ability and a sense of well-being. Nine out of a total of fourteen stated that dance movement therapy had linked feelings to symptoms. Eleven said that it had made them aware of personal needs. Most stated that companionship and belonging to a group had helped considerably.

Areas of improvement were:

- balance
- walking
- handwork
- driving
- the use of feet and ankles
- confidence
- patient's views of partner's attitudes
- carer's opinion of patient
- communication and interaction
- self expression

The aim of the research was to establish that some improvements had been made in particular areas, both physical and psychological. The results showed that benefits to Parkinson's disease patients and their carers focused on the increase in body awareness and an improvement in confidence, which lifted depression. Dance movement therapy does not offer a cure or claim to intervene in Parkinson's disease, but it does offer a support and a means of expressing pain, anger and loss. These emotions affect physical symptoms, as releasing the blocked emotion seems to help. The emotional problems which can interfere with physical abilities can be addressed through the creative medium of dance and movement. This creative medium provides structured activity whereby patterns of movement and behaviour can be repeated and reworked. Through this activity, new possibilities and insights are achieved and assist in the reworking of past experiences so that new patterns of movement evolve and traits of personality are revealed. Parkinson's patients have enabled me to develop patience and sensitivity and, even though at times it has felt like I have been working in death's garden, I have seen many moments that remind me that the human body, when it dances or moves, carries with it the breath of life and the hope that loss and depression can be the wellsprings of a new beginning.

References

Ayres, A.J. (with assistance from J. Robbins) (1991) *Sensory Integration and the Child*. Los Angeles: Western Psychological Services.

Bainbridge Cohen, B. (1993) 'The experiential anatomy of body–mind centering', in *An Introduction to Body–Mind Centering: Sensing, Feeling and Action*. Northampton, Mass.: Contact Editions, pp. 1–6.

Bartenieff, I. (with D. Lewis) (1980) *Body Movement: Coping with the Environment*. New York, Paris, London: Gordon & Breach Science Publishers.

Bull, P.E. (1987) 'The significance of posture, gesture and social interaction'. International Series in Experimental Social Psychology, vol. 16: *Posture and Gesture*. Oxford, New York, Beijing, Frankfurt, São Paulo, Sydney, Tokyo, Toronto: Pergamon Press.

Charcot, J.M. (1880) 'Descriptions of Parkinson's disease', in *De La Paralysie Agitans: Lecons sur les Maladies du Systems Neveux* [Paralysis Agitans, Lessons on Nervous Illnesses]. Paris: Adrian Delahaye, pp. 439–467.

Crickmay, C. and Tufnell, M. (1990) *Body, Space Image*. London: Dance Books.

Gancher, S.T., Hammerstad, J.P. and Nutt, J.G. (1992) 'Parkinson's disease: diagnosis, drug therapy, non-pharmacological interventions', in *Parkinson's Disease: A Hundred Maxims*. London, Melbourne, Auckland: Edward Arnold, Hodder and Stoughton, pp. 10–153.

Hodgkinson, J. (1994) 'The use of stories, role play and fantasy in dementia care', *Journal of Dementia Care: The healing magic of stories*, Sept./Oct., 11.

Joseph, B. and Young, R. (1992) 'The premorbid personality of patients with Parkinson's disease', in B. Joseph and R. Young (eds) *Movement Disorders in Neurology and Psychiatry*. Boston: Blackwell, p. 233.

Kestenberg, J. (1975) *Children and Parents, Psychoanalytic Studies in Development*. New York: Jason Aronson.

Laban, R. (1960) *The Mastery of Movement* (2nd edition, rev. by L. Ullmann). London: MacDonald and Evans Ltd.

Laban, R. and Lawrence, F.C. (1974) *Effort* (2nd edition). London: MacDonald and Evans Ltd.

Lamb, W. (1965) *Posture and Gesture*. London: Gerald Duckworth.

Loman, S. (1990) 'An introduction to the Kestenberg movement profile', in P. Lewis and S. Loman (eds) *The Kestenberg Movement Profile: Its Past, Present Applications and Future Directions*. Keene, N.H.: Antioch New England Graduate School, pp. 52–64.

Marsden, C.D. (1994) 'A full description of Parkinson's disease', *Journal of Neurology, Neurosurgery and Psychiatry* 57: 672–681.

Montagu, A. (1971) *Touching: The Human Significance of the Skin*. New York: Columbia University Press.

North, M. (1972) *Personality through Movement*. London: MacDonald and Evans Ltd.

Parkinson, J. ([1817] 1992) 'An essay on the shaking palsy'. London: Macmillan Magazines Ltd., in association with the Parkinson's Disease Society.

Quinn, N. (1990) 'The 'on–off' phenomenon – the fluctuating response to levodopa'. The On–Off Phenomenon European Conference on Parkinson's Disease and Extrapyramidal Disorders, Rome, 10–14 July.

Sacks, O. (1991) *Awakenings* (rev. edn). London: Pan Books Ltd.

Schore, A.N. (1994) *Affect Regulation and the Origin of the Self*. Hillsdale, N.J.: Lawrence Erlbaum Associates Inc.

Standal, S. (1954) 'The need for positive regard; a contribution to client-centered theory'. Doctoral dissertation, University of Chicago.

Todd, M.E. (1937) *The Thinking Body*. Brooklyn, N.Y.: Dance Horizons Incorporated.

Winnicott, D.W. (1953) 'Transitional objects and transitional phenomena', *International Journal of Psychoanalysis* 34: 89–97.

Chapter 4

Art therapy in the treatment of chronic invalidating conditions

From Parkinson's disease to Alzheimer's

Attilia Cossio

I have worked as an art therapist for several years with patients suffering from chronic invalidating conditions: in particular with adults and elderly people with Parkinson's disease and Alzheimer's. My initial purpose was to offer these patients some moments of well-being and pleasure in a serene and relaxing environment, allowing for artistic activity to perform its cathartic and liberating effect. Later I was able to offer a more focused approach, deriving from the process of painful liberation, compensated by times of intense consolation, which is afforded by a creative act.

A chronic and invalidating disease, treated with drugs that do not cure, in its slow and painful unfolding brings about social isolation accompanied by a deep sense of inadequacy and loss. This is often so severe that patients fall into a state of depression which further inhibits and isolates them.

How then can art therapy be made available to help and support these patients? I would begin to answer this question with the title of one of my recent lectures: 'When drugs are not enough and words are useless . . .'

When drugs treat but do not cure, when words are no consolation, if one loves art one can resort to metaphor, symbols, utterly honest, utterly personal, intimate and sometimes secret and unintelligible even for the person who makes them. As the art process unfolds, the artist is faced with new states of awareness, answers that come from the outside world (that is, other people within the group, the therapist, family members, the therapeutic team . . .) and such answers bring further modification and interaction.

The role of the therapist, in this unfolding of life experiences, is of a delicate nature: encouraging, like a 'good mother', the therapist supports the patient in his or her labour. Like a mother, the therapist observes and 'recognises' in the work the artist and his or her labour, fosters the creative process until the work itself is accomplished, welcomes and encourages the development of relationships. The therapist knows that each work can contain an expression of the person's most secret desires and paramount needs.

In each therapeutic situation we find the cathartic and liberating effect of art therapy and the opportunity to bring to the surface, through symbols and metaphors, the innermost contents of each human experience.

I have chosen to work with people who had no previous art training. It is important that they wanted to have the experience, so they felt the activity to be positive through the discovery of new resources at a time when their life had seemed utterly out of control. Instead it turned into an adventure in which new interests and an opportunity to gain deeper knowledge of the self were acquired.

It is especially interesting to note the value of certain emotional aspects which are present and significant in all patients' work, although their diseases may differ. The first of these is the pleasure felt in seeking beauty and harmony. Beauty and the search for beauty make the fatigue implied in the creative act bearable. We love beauty at all times in our lives, and can achieve it in different ways, for there are many different moments and opportunities to express it. Beauty is always the goal one aims to achieve: it is a reward and a consolation. This is true of healthy people as well as those who are ill but still mentally unaffected, and finally of patients who have lost most of their rational thinking processes.

For example: an elderly woman with Alzheimer's disease, looking once more at a work accomplished during a session, kept whispering to herself (and she never would talk except when at the studio): 'Beautiful . . . beautiful . . . I made this!'

While she concentrated on that painting, another member of the group, also suffering from dementia, looked at her and told me: 'She's old, but the light in her eyes makes her beautiful. Very beautiful!'

It is worth while to note that this remark, amidst a hundred other half-expressed thoughts, reveals an unimpaired sensitivity and an intuition that dementia cannot easily destroy. Art and the pleasure of beauty allow for such revelations.

The second element, directly related to the first, lies in the moment of liberation of emotions, feelings and thoughts. While thoughts which are con-flicted and painful are typically repressed so as not to hurt or annoy others, or because we fear a misunderstanding, they may be released and become socially acceptable thanks to aesthetic transformation and to the poetics of the artistic metaphor.

Another example: at the studio, a woman who had recently suffered a stroke foresaw in a work her imminent death. She had been observing a romantic photograph depicting the sun setting on the sea, in sweet and nuanced colours, and had expressed the wish to reproduce the same atmosphere. While painting, though, she had let herself go to an entirely different rhythm of composition: the sea looked rough and a ship appeared on the horizon, near the left margin of the sheet as if it was about to leave it altogether. The change in style and colours, as compared with her usual way of working, and the fact that she had painted her subject almost without being aware of it, troubled her. With the work group, we celebrated that sort of premonitory dream, turning it into a moment of moving poetry, recalling the ship of dreams in Fellini's film: *E la nave va* . . .

The third important element to be taken into account is the reality of the working group that becomes a support group, with all the interactions and dynamics unfolding along a common pathway. The characteristic feature of art therapy is defined by the fact that expressive activities are substituted for words. This does not mean that we don't also speak, but simply that the dominant language is that of signs, colours and chiaroscuro (light and shade). The language of art is more elusive but no less meaningful than that of words as it leaves a visible trace that can be elaborated in its meanings, for as long as the author needs, in order for possible contents to surface. The author's defences must, however, be fully respected at all times. Nevertheless, the working group emphasises the values of sharing, of interpersonal learning, while the art therapist tries to foster hope and cohesion, the welcoming of each member by another.

A further important element to emphasise concerns the treatment of depression affecting the chronically ill, which is the most immediate consequence of the sense of impotence arising from the loss of health and self-sufficiency. Every project for rehabilitation and treatment must include an enhancement of the individual's creative self, which is why art therapy can be used effectively to counteract and fight forms of depression deriving from invalidating conditions.

For as long as a balance is preserved between the aspects of being and those of doing, it is still possible to work at the removal of the psychological causes of malaise, and the person is then allowed to produce what he or she needs to feel better. Such action is sometimes so effective that positive changes are brought about in the individual's overall tone, with improvements even in the symptoms of the disease. The improvement in self-esteem, the fact that creative abilities and thus the healthy part of the individual are activated, brings about a process of consolidation and re-harmonisation.

Art therapy and Parkinson's disease

I started a trial experience of art therapy for patients suffering from Parkinson's disease in Monza, Italy in 1993, and since then the group has continued meeting at set intervals. A further group was then set up in Milan. With Parkinson's, tremors, rigidity and movement disorders are the most evident physical manifestations. In subtle and invasive fashion, the rigidity of limbs blocks all movement, 'gluing' the patients' feet to the floor, to the point where they cannot lift one to take a step forward. Their voices are altered, food is difficult to swallow, facial expressions absent and inert. Others experience tremors which can affect a side of the body or a limb. Such symptoms are caused by lack of dopamine. As drugs only allow for temporary relief of symptoms, it is important to establish support services to prevent social isolation and provide stimulation, to counteract the rapid degeneration which is the outcome of the disease and to keep the patient as self-sufficient as possible.

Besides the overall aims of art therapy, there are some specific ones which help to foster new experiences and emotions, offer pleasure in quiet and relaxed surroundings, develop a conversational tone, stimulating and giving support.

The great psychological unease of Parkinson's patients cannot be fully soothed, but once faced, the person may come to accept the disease and the unease itself. This is no easy task, as Parkinson's patients are vigilant in their thinking and their intellectual faculties are unimpaired, usually only declining at the advanced stage of the disease and as a consequence of complications. On the other hand, sensitivity and perception are enhanced. Hence the need to achieve a way of consciously living one's dramatic condition with as much serenity as possible, day by day, and to accept the changes that come.

The sense of frustration that leads to depressive states may be mediated through creative activity. Support must continue as long as each person needs it, with appropriate interruptions but also with sufficient consistency to meet the pace and needs of each one.

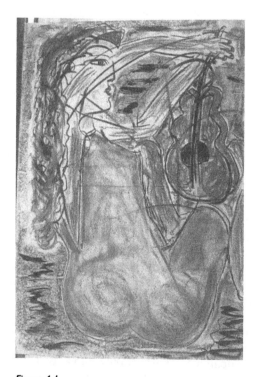

Figure 4.1

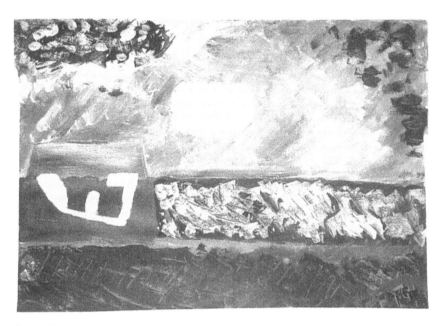

Figure 4.2

In our art therapy studio we have made space for the technique of water-colour. Bright and transparent materials foster a sense of lightness. Laying out colours on wet paper allows the patient to search for and achieve rhythmical gestures, which are especially relaxing and which accompany, as colours on the sheet, the unfolding of thoughts, emotions and reflections. We have also made space for other techniques and materials. Our weekly discussions with the patients emphasise discoveries, the surfacing of insecurities, rebellions and different states of mind. We learn to recognise and accept them. The methodological approach followed is that of my training school (Il Porto) in Turin, Italy. It allows patients to live their own experience in their own way, and to express the psychological movements originating in or following each work. In perceiving the sense of pleasure or pain they derive from their art works, one can devise an approach for subsequent ones.

I also emphasise the unique and unpredictable value of individual resources, the originality of each person's language and the contribution each can offer to the group, so that each emotion has both an exquisitely personal aspect and a social dimension. From the awareness of belonging to a group of ill people we move on to the perception, progressively becoming certainty, of belonging to a group with its own language, codes and interests much beyond the disease itself, and thereby actually bring individuals back to a state of normality.

We have also organised two exhibitions, in public galleries, of works by Parkinson's patients belonging to the art therapy studio in Monza. Such events are not necessary, but represent an interesting opportunity to establish new relations. They have strengthened the self-esteeem and well-being that the groups already show during their activities.

Art therapy and Alzheimer's disease

In early 1996 I organised art therapy workshops for the elderly at the Redaelli Geriatric Institute in Vimodrone, Milan, which includes a Regional Centre for Alzheimer's. One of the first three people in my group was a woman suffering from Alzheimer's.

The title of a congress, held at the Redaelli Institute in September 1996, was: 'The Mystery of Silence' – the silence of patients progressively and inexorably shutting themselves up, taking leave of the world and of all communication. We asked ourselves if the altered behaviour of people with Alzheimer's dementia was solely due to cerebral lesions, or, if read within a psychological frame, might also be understood as symptoms of a mechanism of compensation and escape. A patient who perceives a gradual deconstruction of his or her self, who is losing all traces of his or her past existence, tends to isolate him or herself within an autistic world affording defensive shelter from those feelings of inadequacy and impotence that would be too painful to bear.

In Alzheimer's patients we witness the decay of those faculties which, in analytical terms, are ascribed to the superego. We see the self become fragile and the id become all-pervading. In other words, we witness the choking of reason in favour of instinctual behaviour. While the cortex is less and less able to process thought into abstract concepts, the archipallium, the most ancient part of the human brain and probably the closest to the unconscious, becomes activated.

Non-pharmacological treatments tried up to now are aimed at slowing down the degeneration of cognitive performance and bringing about moments of well-being by working on residual potentialities. We asked ourselves whether such aims could be achieved through artistic activities. Such activities would not be possible without the use of reason and of will. Still, they promote and use the language of the unconscious and that primitive part of thought that is first imagination and then intuition. The patient creates a work, stimulated by a pleasure principle that derives from the achievement of an aesthetic form, gathers a response which is supportive of self because it came about as a result of his or her abilities (creative thought and decision-making first, and then manual ability) which made the work possible (Cossio et al., 1996).

The first aims we set for ourselves in planning the Alzheimer's Nucleus were: offer pleasure, make it possible for patients to relax, stimulate emotions and memories, bring about enhancement of a sense of identity, and positively alter inappropriate behaviour. The method we used to start up communication with Alzheimer's patients was based on empathy; the language used was simple and affectionate. Messages of welcome can be conveyed by facial and vocal expressions, in body gestures communicating in a veritable dance of affection.

There is no healing fantasy for those who work for these patients, and it is impossible to hope to offer them anything more than a little pleasure. Still, it is possible to enhance their abilities, potentialities and emotions, which serves the purpose of redesigning the boundaries of a confused and dimming self. All this seems to be useful, as patients participating in art therapy activities usually show some improvement in language, in the participation in work group events and in a stronger self-awareness.

While all that in the past gave meaning to the life of each of these patients has now relinquished its place to an indistinct and dimmed bundle, we try to establish new and meaningful relations. We reveal residual abilities that often could not have been unveiled in any other way; we activate channels of communication that unfold a concealed world of affections, and even when the artistic expression seems poor it still unveils the uniqueness of hidden individual worlds.

Responses to the stimulation of the art therapist differ from patient to patient. Some need the therapist to act as a very supportive friend; they ask for constant support and help, for containment to the extent that the boundaries of the self appear confused. Some ask for the pleasure of moving about

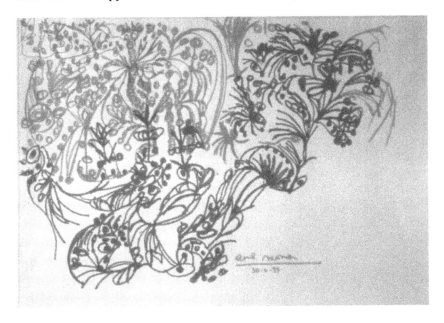

Figure 4.3

in freedom among colours that become places of pleasure to be enjoyed like food (and often they are truly 'tasted'). In these cases the art therapist must contain outbursts and destructiveness, so that each work will be preserved in its wholeness and bear witness to the creative act that has taken place. The artist signs the work with a signature he or she will recognise even in the near future, though memory may fail.

Patients at the Alzheimer's Nucleus are typically suffering from probable Alzheimer's, with severe dementia. One woman enjoys painting but uses the brush like a pencil to draw in colours. At the beginning of her stay in hospital she suffered from persecution fantasies, with visual hallucinations. When taken to the studio she was very restless, and was not undergoing pharmacological treatment. She could never draw straight lines. Her compositions were very pleasant, much admired by friends, and others are arabesques representing the mazes of the mind from which the faces of little friendly gnomes emerge. In her painting she has evoked real events and people in her life that she had never revealed before to anyone at the hospital.

Another woman was eventually able to cry while unconsciously drawing

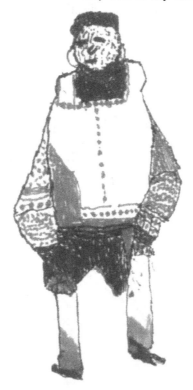

Figure 4.4

teardrops on a face she had painted, though she had said she never cried over the pain she had endured in her life.

Another woman can draw human figures from which fragments of her past surface into memory, and despite being 90 she dreams like an 18-year-old girl.

As in dreams, artistic production opens a window on to those lands where each person's life story has taken place. The therapist adapts to the inclinations and specific situation of each patient, trying to emphasise all the good results and compensate for times of unease. Each message is received and conveyed through analogical form and through the language of affection. The choice of materials is made on the basis of their symbolic values and of the psychological needs expressed. While we approve of special techniques and results, first and foremost we perceive the pleasure of restoring for our patients a deep sense of their own dignity.

Reference

Cossio, A., Sacco, S., Scalisi, P., Casale, G. (1996) 'Images from silence'. 3rd Congress on Alzheimer's Disease, Budapest, Hungary.

Chapter 5

Case studies in Huntington's disease

Music therapy assessment and treatment in the early to advanced stages[1]

Wendy L. Magee

The ideas presented in this chapter are a reflection of the author's experience over a five-year period working with people living with Huntington's disease (HD). During this period, different approaches were explored to find those which offered maximum support to clients in their differing stages of the condition. Approaches employed needed constant re-evaluation, as HD is typified by a gradual change in abilities over an extended period of deterioration. A definition and description of the symptoms of HD are given, followed by behaviours and responses observed in music therapy sessions presented in case study format.

Definition and description of Huntington's disease

Huntington's disease is a chronic, progressive, hereditary disease affecting the central nervous system, stemming from damage to the basal ganglia within the brain. It causes motor, cognitive and emotional disorders in the affected individual, and although the average age of onset is 36–45 years of age, symptoms may begin at any time of the affected person's life, from childhood to old age (Folstein, 1989). It is an autosomal dominant disorder, meaning each child born to a parent with the HD gene has a 50 per cent chance of also carrying the gene and developing the disease. It is not HD which causes death for the affected person; secondary illnesses, such as pneumonia or cardio-respiratory illness, have been found to be the most common causes of death (Harper, 1991; Folstein, 1989).

The illness is characterised by involuntary movements and abnormality of voluntary movements, gradual deterioration of certain cognitive skills, and emotional disorders causing complex social consequences for the individual and their family or support network.

Movement problems may involve large, 'choreic' movements or cause rigidity and slowness involving arms, legs, fingers, trunk, neck, head and face. Speech becomes dysrhythmic, occurring in bursts with pauses in mid-phrase, and also slower and dysarthric, causing the listener difficulty in interpreting the spoken message. Difficulty in initiating speech causes considerable delay in responding verbally to even a simple request or command. Swallowing problems develop, and in the later stages the use of direct feeding methods such as nasogastric tube or gastrostomy may be necessary to ensure adequate nutrition.

Early cognitive symptoms are likely to involve memory problems and an inability to organise information, and progressively result in decreased abilities in problem-solving, initiation, and concentration. The individual will experience increasing difficulty in verbal expression, the ability to change from one task to another, retrieval of information and memories, and the speed with which they can process information and act on it. There is a marked loss of spontaneity and a reduced ability to participate in novel situations. Conscious related functions such as knowing and insight, however, may be relatively well preserved even into the most advanced stages of the illness (Shoulson, 1990).

Psychiatric disorders associated with HD may be seen years before motor or cognitive symptoms have caused the illness to be diagnosed, resulting in distress and often stigma for the affected individual and their family. Depression, irritability and apathy are the most often exhibited symptoms, with other psychiatric conditions such as schizophrenic symptoms, delusional disorders, mania and anxiety commonly being seen (Folstein, 1989; Morris, 1991). Behavioural problems and personality changes caused by emotional disorder may include sexual inappropriateness, aggressive behaviour, suicidal tendencies, and drug and alcohol abuse. The psychosocial effects on the individual, their spouse, children and support network can be tremendously complicated.

Literature review

A review of the research and descriptive literature reveals that music therapy is particularly beneficial as part of music and movement programmes (Rainey Perry, 1983; Groom and Dawes, 1985), relaxation programmes (Rainey Perry, 1983), or to facilitate speech through singing (Erdonmez, 1976; Hoskyns, 1981; Rainey Perry, 1983). Music therapy also may act as a catalyst for discussion and emotional expression through songwriting or by encouraging the group or individual to choose songs with themes or lyrics with which they identify (Curtis, 1987; Dawes, 1985a, 1985b). This last technique, described as 'counselling-oriented music therapy', appears to be relevant when working with people in the early or advanced stages of HD, justifying it as an attractive and useful therapeutic tool when working with a client over a long period of time. This is particularly so considering that other media and activities usually become unrealistic or impossible for the client to participate in as they become increasingly disabled.

Judging from the literature, it would certainly seem that using familiar songs offers a more easily measurable activity for research or evaluation pur-poses in therapy programmes, particularly important in the current climate of proving 'effectiveness' to service purchasers. However, the use of instru-mental improvisation is only briefly described (Hoskyns, 1981), and leaves a question as to what the benefits are of this activity with this population, particularly considering the certainty of increasing physical debility and the likelihood of cognitive degeneration.

Music therapy as part of a treatment programme

Music therapy can be seen to offer a range of experiences which may be denied to the person in their everyday life due to the physical, communication and cognitive changes they are experiencing.

Even when large choreic movements or minimal movements become impossible because rigidity render functional tasks impossible, playing musical instruments provides a purpose for attempting exploration of the environment. For clients with large, uncontrolled voluntary movements, using instruments with a large surface area – such as bass xylophones or large-headed drums and cymbals – optimises success in achieving a sound for the often enormous effort involved. For those with minimal rigid move-ments, the use of instruments suspended on a stand, such as triangle or windchimes, positioned close to the hand allows independence in achieving feedback for the involved effort. Other instruments provide maintenance and development of fine motor skills, such as the use of keyboard, or strumming instruments which involve fine finger movements or the manipulation of a plectrum. Encouraging decision-making through offering a choice of instrument is considered to be an added creative and expressive component to exploration of the environment, particularly when there may be few areas in their life where the client is still able or allowed to express choice or make decisions.

As speech becomes increasingly difficult for others to understand, and the content of speech repetitive and 'stuck' or seemingly meaningless, it is likely that attempting any verbal communication is a highly frustrating experience for the client. Music-making, either through singing or instrumental playing, can alleviate this to some extent by providing opportunities for recognition of the individual and creative expression through a non-verbal medium.

As the individual experiences difficulty in communicating, changes in behaviour, and changes in their physical abilities, they are likely to become increasingly isolated. Maintaining regular employment becomes more dif-ficult, and the individual may become increasingly self-conscious about their 'abnormal' behaviour. Opportunities for socialising decrease, and relation-ships with family and friends are often affected. The opportunity to build meaningful relationships with others, which may be severely impaired in usual settings, may be possible in a music therapy setting. This can be the case particularly for people who have had an active background in music-making or appreciation.

Lastly, music-making can act as a powerful motivator even when the person's ability to initiate other activities is impaired.

Music therapy in the early stages of HD

In the early stages of the illness, the person living with HD is likely to be maintaining a semblance of an independent lifestyle, still living in their own home, and possibly still employed. Physical symptoms may not be causing serious disability; however, they will be noticeable in the affected person's walking pattern, facial expression, and on attempting any task. Commonly, cognitive changes cause problems with short-term memory and tasks which require the abilities to organise, calculate, or carry out complex processes. The individual may experience behavioural or psychiatric changes causing bizarre, unreasonable, or aggressive behaviour which seriously affects the spouse or children living with them, and can result in marital breakdown. Emotional lability, confusion and social withdrawal are the most commonly reported responses to the dramatic changes occurring in the affected individual (Tyler, 1991).

The picture of the person living in the early stages of the illness, therefore, is one of increasing isolation and emotional turmoil as the individual attempts to adjust to the changes happening to them. If insight is impaired, they may be experiencing confusion as to why situations around them do not make sense, or why others are behaving in such an inexplicable way, telling them what to do. Previous occupations or pastimes gradually become impossible due to the physical changes occurring, communicating with speech becomes increasingly frustrating, and the possibility of experiencing something novel or pleasurable appears greatly diminished.

In the author's experience, clients at this stage may benefit from individual rather than group therapy, giving them the space to take risks and time to reflect on how they are feeling or what they are experiencing. Placing clients in a group can be difficult, as being with other HD clients at different stages can be confronting and painful as they view where they will 'end up'. Placing the client in a group with people with other conditions can also be problematic if it heightens their isolation when other group members are intolerant of the HD client's difficulty in communicating, or find their choreic movements disturbing.

The main aim of the session may be to engage the client in a musical activity by focusing on the creative and expressive qualities of the music, attempting to use less-structured music such as instrumental improvisation where possible. The client is encouraged to explore as widely as possible, in terms of instrument choice and musical style, although their right to express a constant preference is respected. All tasks involve active participation, and the music therapist needs to assess continually the client's ability to organise information, remember previous material, interact musically, and the tendency to perseverate on material. The therapist aims to draw out the client's strengths in the sessions, and to work towards maintaining and developing these. Areas which need particular consideration include the client's ability to initiate change, which can affect their ability to stop playing at the end of a musical activity or change from one activity to another, as perseverative mannerisms in the music may continue from one task to the next. Memory deficits combined with an inability to stop playing may cause turn-taking activities to be inappropriate, as even simple instructions are not retained or followed. Using familiar songs, the music therapy session may provide a safe environment in which to vocalise, which may be becoming increasingly difficult in other situations.

Case study: 'Joseph'

'Joseph', a man in his mid-forties with HD, was referred to music therapy on his admission to a day care facility, having been recently diagnosed. He was reported to be experiencing changing behaviour due to his illness, and increasing isolation, compounded by an 'uncertain future'. He was still ambulant, although he walked with large swaying movements, and any intentional movement in his arms was clumsy and jerky due to ataxia. His speech was slurred, and the content perseverative, often being repetitive and limited in variation. He was reported to have moderately impaired memory, and had started to exhibit some delusional beliefs. When referred to music therapy, the team hoped that it would provide an 'emotional outlet and means of expression' for him, as his verbal communication appeared limited. He had no previous musical experience.

In 16 months of attending music therapy sessions, Joseph stated that he enjoyed sessions, and appeared to gain confidence in his new-found skill. Activities had centred around instrument playing, largely in improvisation with the therapist.

He expressed a preference in each session for the metallophone and the electric piano on 'pipe organ' mode, and appeared to have some difficulty in exploring more than one instrument per session, tending to stay on the first chosen one unless prompted to change. Unless activities had a definite beginning and ending, such as a song-based activity, he had difficulty stopping playing when the music ended, appearing to rely on visual prompts such as the therapist changing body posture away from the instrument. He was able to repeat only the simplest rhythms given, such as three or four crotchet beats, and when given a more complex pattern would return the correct number of sounds played but with no rhythmic organisation (i.e. six quavers and a crotchet would be repeated as seven 'sounds'). This was felt to be due to a combination of difficulty with organising the information and problems with co-ordination, as if the given pulse was kept slow he was able to repeat it with greater accuracy. He also had difficulty participating in turn-taking activities, being unable to stop playing in each of his turns, although this reduced somewhat if the therapist was sharing the same instrument. Generally he became completely engrossed in his own playing and appeared to have little awareness of the therapist's music regardless of dramatic dynamic, rhythmic or harmonic variations. His playing on the two chosen instruments involved repeated descending and ascending scales, or repeated playing of small areas on an instrument, such as three notes descending on the piano or metallophone, or three or four strings on the autoharp or guitar, despite being physically able to reach the full range.

Overall, his playing showed a marked lack of spontaneity, with repeated patterns from which he seemed unable to depart, and a tendency to organise his playing spatially.

The changes which gradually emerged during the treatment period included becoming more aware of the end of a piece of music, particularly the familiar 'welcome chant' in which he started to anticipate the end. He also extended his playing of the keyboard to use two hands, although he remained unable to co-ordinate his movements to do this with the metallophone. The patterns he played on the keyboard expanded from simple scales to more complex ones combining sustained notes and slow trills or leaping intervals of fourths or thirds using both hands; however, these appeared to become as perseverative in nature as the scale patterns. In the last few weeks of the 16-month treatment period his playing became much louder, more energetic, and broke away more from his repetitive patterns. However, his playing continued to lack spontaneity in reaction to the therapist's music. This dramatic change in his playing occurred at a time when a change in his living environment caused him to confront the painful reality of his illness, causing aggressive outbursts at home. The team felt that in his music he was starting to express the many difficult feelings which he was unable to express verbally.

Music therapy in the middle stage of HD

People in the middle stages of the illness may still be ambulant, although have increasing difficulty maintaining their balance. It is more likely that a wheelchair is necessary. Choreic movements become more obvious, and the individual is more dependent for overall care. Communication is severely impaired, as speech is poorly articulated, inappropriate in content, or may occur only in bursts. If cognitive skills allow, the person may be able to use a communication aid, although this would also be dependent on their willingness to use it. Poor initiation can affect speech and behaviour in general, requiring an immense amount of time for a delayed response to even a simple request. Cognitive deficits may come into play here as well, as the person may have increasing difficulty organising and processing information, concentrating on tasks presented, or remembering instructions given. Behaviour may be generally unpredictable, and requests can result in an absence of response, refusal to comply, or in angry or aggressive outbursts.

In the author's experience, group treatment can be beneficial with the person in the middle stages of the illness, as this allows for a natural 'time out' from activities when there are lapses in attention or concentration. Group activities can also give the client the amount of time needed for their delayed responses, using others' turns as a prompt or visual model of the activity. Choice-making may be the focus of tasks at this stage, particularly with instruments which can be chosen without the need for speech. Music, whether for instrumental activities or singing, needs to be highly structured to facilitate organisation of information, either using familiar songs, improvisations based on familiar melodies, or tasks where there is a gap within the musical framework for making sounds on an instrument. The framework provided by familiar songs can also aid clients who have memory deficits, and can facilitate more spontaneous participation for those with initiation difficulties. Songs are also particularly useful for those who no longer have functional speech, encouraging verbalisation of well-rehearsed lines. Alternatively, activities may remain non-verbal in the form of instrument playing.

Case study: 'Caroline'

'Caroline' was a 50-year-old woman who was hospitalised when her living situation was considered to place her at risk of danger, no longer being able to care for herself or organise her daily activities. This was also complicated by her living with immediate family members who were thought to be showing early behavioural symptoms of HD. On admission to the hospital she was very withdrawn and refused to participate in any form of activity by becoming verbally aggressive. Her contact with music therapy began with occasional attendance of a group with other HD clients who were in more advanced stages of the disease.

She later started to attend another music therapy group with people who had other conditions, and hence different types of abilities and difficulties. Her speech was nearly impossible to understand due to dysarthria, and she had impaired awareness of others, resulting in poor social skills. Because of this she initially received mixed reactions from the others in the group who could all speak clearly and had trouble understanding why she did not respond verbally to their greetings and other interactions. She was, however, highly responsive to the instruments, and expressed great pleasure through her facial gestures during instrumental activities which helped the others in the group to warm in their interactions with her. Although her memory and cognition could not be assessed by conventional neuropsychological tests, her behaviour in the music therapy group suggested that she was carrying material over from one week to the next, indicated by her recall of the welcome song and her precision in choosing a different instrument to play each week.

Because Caroline's speech was severely impaired she rarely spoke; however, she often sang to familiar songs, particularly the welcome song and other very familiar songs which were discovered to be favourites. The emphasis for her in the group was on non-verbal activities, particularly on choosing instruments, as this was something over which she took a great deal of time and did very thoughtfully. Instrument playing appeared to give her an enormous amount of pleasure, causing her to become animated, which was in stark contrast to her behaviour in other settings when she tended to sit still and interacted very little with the surrounding environment.

Problems which arose and needed to be worked around included her very delayed physical and verbal responses to questions or requests, which meant that the rest of the group had to wait for the time she needed to choose an instrument, partner or song. Presenting a limited choice of instruments with only visual prompts and instrumental sounds appeared to make the process of choosing easier for her than using verbal instructions. Turn-taking activities were not appropriate due to the complexity of the instructions and her difficulty in stopping playing and 'passing a turn' to the next person. Often actions or instructions needed to be broken down into steps to facilitate processing of the information and serve as a prompt. The use of familiar music in structured activities appeared to enable her to participate to her maximum level of functioning and respond more spontaneously.

Through her enthusiasm and interest in playing Caroline gradually became more popular within the group, who appeared to become more accepting of her non-verbal participation. Whilst music was kept familiar and tasks involved instrument playing, she was able to participate to her maximum level of ability.

Music therapy in the advanced stages

The individual in the advanced stages of the illness is likely to be completely dependent for all aspects of care, and to have severely reduced opportunities for participating in any activity other than passively. Due to the high level of care needed by the individual, the family may choose to place the affected person into hospital care. By this stage, feeding by conventional methods may have been replaced by alternative methods such as gastrostomy or nasogastric feeding, and communication may be only through indication of 'yes/no' or completely absent. Choreic movements may render all functional or voluntary activity impossible, and be very disturbing to observe for family or those who are unfamiliar with the disease. Movements are most probably constant, only ceasing during sleep, and the individual requires an enormous calorie intake – 5,000 each day – to obtain adequate nutrition for the amount of energy being used.

It is important that the therapist structures all activities around the client's remaining skills when working with people in the advanced stages of HD. Clients may still be able to turn their heads intentionally or gaze towards a specific target, be able to communicate 'yes/no' by pointing to communication cards, or be able to play instruments which give good feedback for minimal or rigid movements. It is unlikely that intentional vocalisation remains at this stage.

For clients in the advanced stages, group treatment is recommended, focusing on the individual for their turn within each activity, giving the others in the group a break from attending to tasks. Music which has been found to be the most beneficial in keeping participants' attention are very familiar popular songs or pieces of well-known classical music, or improvisations structured on familiar tunes. Songs which include the participants' names, as part of welcome or goodbye activities, are particularly useful in helping to maintain a participant's attention, and keep them orientated to the group. If a participant can still turn their head, this may be incorporated into a welcome activity, where they can turn to look at another member of the group to pass on the 'hello'. Music which has been a particular favourite in the past can be discovered by talking to family members, and can be introduced to the group as having a special meaning for the person involved. Although the therapist makes every effort to use live music which has been found to be more stimulating than taped, it is not always possible to reproduce particular pieces, hence taped music might be used.

Large, involuntary choreic movements may render all intentional movement impossible, in which case passive or receptive techniques may be more suitable. These may involve the use of tactile instruments such as the autoharp or guitar positioned unobtrusively on a part of the body, or guided imagery combined with instructed deep-breathing exercises. If functional or intentional movement exists, however, active instrument playing may be possible. Participants may be able to choose an instrument from a very limited choice offered (i.e. two only at a time), either by positioning the instruments clearly to the left or right of the participant and asking them to look towards their choice, or by presenting only one instrument at a time and using 'yes/no' cards if this is the client's method of communication. Verbal directions and prompts may need to be replaced by solely visual and auditory presentation of the instruments. This may help to reduce the complexity of the task overall. Preference for a particular instrument can be gauged over time and included in the initial choice offered each time. This type of decision-making can be a focus of the group, facilitating active participation for even the most disabled.

Finally, the family may be involved, particularly when the affected person is at this stage. There may be few occasions where a family member may observe the affected person being actively and purposely involved in a leisure activity, and few opportunities for them to share something meaningful together. The music therapy session can offer a chance to express humour or sadness within a contained, supportive environment. Although the techniques outlined here highlight the severe disability of the population, the opportunity actively to engage in music-making or decision-making cannot be dismissed lightly when it may be the only chance these clients have to do so.

Case study: 'Ted'

'Ted' was a man in his fifties living on the HD unit of the hospital, and was completely dependent for all aspects of daily living, having only minimal rigid movements. He remained sufficiently cognitively intact to use a simple communication board and to respond to simple questions, and particularly to humour which had always been a strong part of his personality. His communication board was very limited, having 'yes', 'no', and several other functional words written on it, to which he pointed using his finger. This meant that when he needed to communicate something, he was dependent on someone presenting him with the board, or if the thing which he wished to communicate was not represented there, dependent on the person being familiar or sensitive enough to guess what he wanted. He had occasional behavioural outbursts, but it was usually difficult to ascertain the immediate reason for these due to his difficulty in communicating. His interaction with others consisted of being attended to by the nurses for his basic needs and visits from his mother, and he mostly stayed in his room watching the television. He had previously been an active sportsman with a wide variety of interests, including playing instruments in a band. He was therefore very isolated, with little opportunity for interacting with others or actively participating in a meaningful activity.

Ted attended a music therapy group for 4–6 people in the advanced stage of HD. His active participation consisted of being able to choose the next person in the 'hello' activity by looking towards the person he chose, and by being able to choose an instrument to play either by looking towards one of a choice of two, or communicating 'yes/no' through his communication board. His favoured instruments included the maracas in both hands and a triangle placed on a stand hanging over him with a lightweight beater. During a 'goodbye improvisation' played each week, Ted made an enormous effort to achieve sounds from his chosen instrument with his very rigid movements, playing deliberately only when his name was sung in the improvisation, indicating a full awareness of events. Songs which had been previous favourites or that he had played in his band were discovered through discussion with his mother, and these were incorporated into an activity which included significant music for each member of the group on alternate weeks. This activity helped to highlight each person as an individual with personal preferences, which was not an easy task in other settings. It also encouraged Ted's mother to be involved in the group, which was one of her only chances to see Ted participating actively in anything, and allowed opportunities for reminiscence and meaningful interactive communication between the two.

Summary

The author believes that music therapy has a vital part to play in a treatment programme over an extended period of time for a person living with HD, throughout the different stages progressively experienced. It is essential, however, that the music therapist be aware of not only the emotional and physical effects of the illness but also take into account the client's cognitive abilities in order to create a music therapy programme which will offer maximum support and facilitate active participation for the client, enhancing their quality of life. This may mean considering the appropriateness of musical forms and structures used, and whether free or structured improvisation, or familiar well-learnt songs, may be most suitable for maintaining the client's engagement.

Note

1 The Royal Hospital of Neuro-disability received a proportion of its funding to support this paper from the NHS Executive. The views represented are those of the author, not necessarily of the NHSE. The paper is reproduced by kind permission of the *British Journal of Music Therapy*.

References

Curtis, S. (1987) Music therapy: a positive approach in Huntington's disease. *Proceedings of the 13th National Conference of the Australian Music Therapy Association Incorporated.* Sydney: Australian Music Therapy Association Inc.

Dawes, S. (1985a) The role of music therapy in caring in Huntington's disease, in E. Chiu and B. Teltscher (eds) *Handbook for Caring in Huntington's Disease,* Melbourne: Huntington's Disease Clinic.

Dawes, S. (1985b) Case study: advanced stage Huntington's disease. *Proceedings of the 11th National Conference of the Australian Music Therapy Association Incorporated.* Sydney: Australian Music Therapy Association Inc., pp. 87–92.

Erdonmez, D. (1976) The effect of music therapy in the treatment of Huntington's chorea patients. *Proceedings of the 2nd National Conference of the Australian Music Therapy Association Incorporated.* Sydney: Australian Music Therapy Association Inc., pp. 58–64.

Folstein, S. (1989) *Huntington's Disease: A Disorder of Families.* London: The Johns Hopkins University Press.

Groom, J. and Dawes, S. (1985) Enhancing the self-image of people with Huntington's disease through the use of music, movement and dance. *Proceedings of the 11th National Conference of the Australian Music Therapy Association Incorporated.* Sydney: Australian Music Therapy Association Inc., pp. 66–67.

Harper, P. (1991) The natural history of Huntington's disease, in P. Harper (ed.) *Huntington's Disease*. London: W.B. Saunders Company Ltd.

Hoskyns, S. (1981) An investigation of the value of music therapy in the care of patients suffering from Huntington's chorea. Unpublished manuscript.

Morris, M. (1991) Psychiatric aspects of Huntington's disease, in P. Harper (ed.) *Huntington's Disease*. London: W.B. Saunders Company Ltd.

Rainey Perry, M. (1983) Music therapy in the care of Huntington's disease patients. *Australian Music Therapy Association Bulletin* December 6(4): 3–10.

Shoulson, I. (1990) Huntington's disease: cognitive and psychiatric features. *Neuropsychiatry, Neuropsychology, and Behavioural Neurology* 3(1): 15–22.

Tyler, A. (1991) Social and psychological aspects of Huntington's disease, in P. Harper (ed.) *Huntington's Disease*. London: W.B. Saunders Company Ltd.

Chapter 6

Art therapy with older adults clinically diagnosed as having Alzheimer's disease and dementia

John Tyler

Introduction

Before I trained as an art therapist I worked as a teacher with children in primary, middle and secondary schools. Art was my specialism, and I noticed how lessons where children were free to express themselves, without being confined to themes, provoked individual and personal imagery. The art they created often appeared to say much about each child's unique inner landscape and experience of the world. It seemed to me that their paintings and drawings spoke for them, and that what they put on paper they might not have been able to articulate verbally.

During my clinical practice, whilst training as an art therapist, I became interested in working with older people. I was on placement in a large Victorian psychiatric hospital, and offered group and individual sessions to older adults. These people were generally depressed as a result of experiencing multiple losses associated with older age. Their artwork frequently appeared to embody their feelings and accompanying emotions. I sensed a relief and release for these people as a result of the art-making process. Similar to my experience with children, these older adults might not have been able to express what they could embody in the image through words.

I currently work as a state registered art therapist in an NHS Trust hospital. Over the past ten years I have offered therapy both on a one-to-one basis and in groups to older adults with a clinical diagnosis of Alzheimer's disease and dementia. My increasing view is that art therapy, being a primarily non-verbal process, offers these people increased control over their lives. As a consequence of the freedom to explore the use of art materials, they have the opportunity to organise their experience in their own way without expectations from others. Despite their cognitive impairments I believe the experience of art therapy for these people can be both healing and liberating.

More recently, whilst pursuing a four-year psychotherapy training, I have become more aware of the breadth and depth of personal transformations that appear to take place in the process I am describing. Consequently, I am interested in exploring the hypothesis that art therapy can assist people experiencing memory loss to resolve significant conflicts during the final stages of life as we know it.

Persona non grata?

Older adults can face considerable losses as they age. These losses include employment, health, mobility, cognition, friends and loved ones, independence, and appetite for life. They begin to feel less useful and they can be treated as if they were 'on the scrap heap'. Although they may be cared for in terms of their physical well-being, there may be little on offer that focuses upon their emotional and psychological welfare.

The culture we live in tends to dismiss older people over retirement age, perhaps suggesting that what they have to offer is of little value. This is probably more marked where people who are experiencing varying degrees of memory loss are concerned. Furthermore, through the concern of their carers they can be treated more like children than adults. They may also act like children if the only part of their memory that is intact connects them with their distant past.

In a care setting, someone experiencing memory loss can feel emotionally isolated and confused about what is happening to them. They may have a strong need to make sense of their situation and have a place where they can freely express their feelings and emotions. Older adults are frequently viewed by society as less attractive and there may be many reasons why carers avoid getting 'too close' to them. In a culture that praises youth and vigour, communicating with older people can bring us in touch with our own ageing process, and perhaps that of our parents. We can begin to examine our own wrinkles and blemishes. In other words, we can get in touch with our mortality and our beliefs about what happens when we die.

Despite the difficulties and challenges of working with older adults suffering memory loss, I believe it is crucial that caregivers avoid treating them as if they no longer understand what is happening around them or to them personally. Some years ago I remember a voluntary worker asking me whether the person I saw for art therapy had done anything in the session that week. This was asked when the person I had been working with was standing beside me. I think this is a good example of the potential for older people with memory loss to be dismissed and written off as if they have nothing to contribute. They can run the risk of being talked about rather than talked to, thereby becoming *persona non grata*. If they are suffering from memory loss they may already be beginning to struggle with their identity and purpose.

Therefore talking about them as if they are not there just confirms and possibly increases their demise.

The question as to whether the person has done something or not is an interesting one in itself and perhaps conveys an attitude towards working with this client group; namely, that it might be a surprise if anything is done or achieved or can be done and achieved in therapy. Older people can frequently be given up on and the last stage of life seen as marking time.

In one setting I used to visit, art activities for older people had been organised in such a way as to ensure results that could then be displayed. Each older person was only involved in a small part of the total process; for example, colouring-in something that had already been outlined by a volunteer. The emphasis of such activity seemed to be on making sure there was a tangible and recognisable result at the end. Perhaps the structure of such exercises had more to do with the needs of the carers than the needs of the older people themselves. Maybe it allowed the carers to feel they had done something constructive that others could see and admire. I noticed that in the spring colourful cut-out daffodils and tulips, spring lambs and Easter chicks would be stuck to walls and windows, and, upon looking at these images, I was quickly reminded of my own early years in primary school. I also knew these displays were created mainly by the staff. In the same setting, other displays would occur throughout the year: Halloween witches on broomsticks, fireworks pictures, valentine hearts, winter snowflakes and the inevitable Christmas trees.

Although carers are generally well meaning, older people suffering varying degrees of confusion and memory loss can be disempowered and treated like children. This in turn may increase dependence, and once the older person becomes used to being treated thus they are likely to do less and less for themselves as a result.

The freedom to be yourself

At the beginning of the first art therapy group I ever facilitated for older adults with memory loss, I remember suggesting it might be a good idea if we began by introducing ourselves. I had no idea that one of the group members had forgotten who they were and could not recall their own name. Memory impairment can vary dramatically from one person to another and is not a static and fixed phenomenon. Someone can be lucid in one moment and totally confused in the next. My way of working, I hope, maximises the opportunity for people freely to create as they wish, if they wish. I will make the art materials readily available but I will not suggest anything to the person in terms of what to do. As a result, whatever occurs is a direct consequence of the individual's own choice.

In my experience, when older people suffering memory loss come to the art therapy room for their first sessions they frequently appear lost and make comments or non-verbal expressions and gestures that suggest they are unfamiliar with the environment. Often it is as if they are experiencing the art therapy session for the very first time, even though they may in fact have been coming for many weeks. The images created by one individual can be almost identical every week, whereas by another completely different each time. The artwork might be symbolically charged, or alternatively a safe tried and tested formula that is experienced as less frightening to create. With repetitive imagery what strikes me is a sense of holding on to something that at some level is familiar. It is always difficult to know why particular images are created and what lies behind them. Frequently the person is unable to convey much verbally about the experience but may repeat the same phrases over and over again, which in time may give some clues.

One woman in her late seventies was referred for art therapy because of her short-term memory loss and impaired verbal communication skills. There was a naive and childlike quality to the way she presented, and I was struck by how readily she agreed to come over to the art therapy room despite the fact that we had never met before. In our first meeting I found myself feeling concerned, as I might for a child who too easily is willing to go off with a stranger, and I immediately felt protective towards her, sensing her vulnerability.

Every week she would come into the art therapy room and, after hanging her coat behind the door, take the same chair and use exactly the same materials to create an almost identical image each time. She never referred to her previous paintings, which were all kept available in a folder on a nearby table with her name boldly printed on the front. When she entered the room it was as if she had never visited before and she would make a comment about how nice it was to be there.

It appeared she thought of herself as a child. She often mentioned her dead mother as if she were still alive and would be worried about not getting home in time for tea. Sometimes she seemed concerned that she hadn't brought any money with her to the session, and would unravel her handkerchief as if expecting to find it there. I wondered with her what she felt she needed the money for. This dialogue between us occurred frequently and she would say in a very disjointed way that the money she had forgotten was either to pay for the art materials or for her dinner. She would worry that her mother would be cross with her for losing it. It was hard for her to accept that she didn't need money to come to art therapy as she did not seem to know where she was.

I wondered if she was relating to me as if I was a teacher and she was at school. I remembered my days of teaching in primary school when the first job on a Monday morning after taking the register was to collect the dinner money. Occasionally she indicated that she thought I had invited her into my own home, and it seemed she felt the art materials personally belonged to me. I tried to convey that the art materials were free of charge and that she had as much right to use them as anyone else. One phrase she managed at the end of each session was 'thank you for having me'. This reminded me of my own childhood as I had been taught to say this to the parents of school friends I went to tea with.

Gradually she became more confident to use the art materials without feeling a need to pay for them. Each week she came and chose a small piece of paper, painting a strip of grass at the bottom and a strip of sky at the top. Like many small children's paintings, there was no horizon and just a void between the sky and the ground. In this space between she painted animals and a barn. Because of her memory loss she found it difficult to string more that a few words together, but each week when she finished painting she would manage a few comments. In this way she began to tell the story of her childhood in weekly instalments. Sometimes she repeated the phrases from a previous week, and sometimes she added something new. I slowly gained from her a picture of her childhood during the war years when she was evacuated to the countryside and lived on a farm. This was a time she had clearly loved and she was so absorbed whilst she was painting it was as if she had literally gone back there to revisit. Her belief that she was living at home with her mother, who always had tea waiting, made me believe she was living in the past. Perhaps in this way she avoided the painful reality that her parents and her husband had all long since died. Perhaps also she wished to be young again and to turn back the clock.

Each time she came she created a similar image to that of the previous

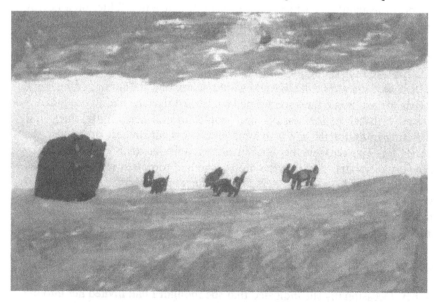

Figure 6.1 For colour versions of figures in this chapter please see
www.brunner-routledge.co.uk/WallerArtsTherapies

week. Hence a series of images were produced which were quite repetitive and identical in their format and execution. An example of this can be found in Figure 6.1. Sky and ground would be disconnected, between which scenes of animals walking towards a barn would be depicted. She would never refer to her previous paintings despite her folder of work being visibly present in the room. The skies were dark blue, perhaps suggesting early evening, and the round yellow orbs suggested moons rather than suns.

Whilst she worked the process took all of her concentration and she seemed completely unaware of the rest of the group. It was as if she was locked into her inner world and had withdrawn from the reality of her physical surroundings. Upon completing the animals she would look up and beam. There was a strong sense of accomplishment as well as relief when she finished each painting, as if something crucially important had been achieved.

One week she came into the room and immediately remarked 'Oh, I've been here before.' This felt like a breakthrough and led me to believe that the continuity of the sessions and the environment allowed her to recapture her memory and therefore gain more control of her life. She was always very pleased with the animals she created and once the brown paint had dried she sometimes added blue eyes, this making her laugh whenever she did it. Her attention when finishing a painting would come back to the room. She became quite animated at these times and loved to hold her painting up for others to see and attempt to say something about her memories of the farm. I felt there was a shrine-like quality about the imagery as it seemed so important for her to repeat it each week, even though at this time it appeared she didn't know she had done it before. The animals were always depicted as if moving towards their resting place, and I wondered about her own life journey.

One day when she had completed her painting she asked about what she called 'the old ones'. I quickly realised she might be talking about her previous images for the very first time. On exploring this with her it became clear she wanted to see her previous paintings. When I presented her with the folder containing her paintings she seemed overjoyed. She explored each of them in turn carefully taking them out of the folder and laying them in front of her on the table. She seemed surprised to see so many.

It was at this point in the therapy, as she inspected her work, that she made the comment 'not finished' in relation to the paintings. Over the following weeks, the exploration of her previous work would always begin the session. She would ask to see 'the old ones' and would then select a painting to continue with. She would concentrate on filling in the void between the sky and the ground by bringing down the skyline until it met the grass, and in this way create a horizon (see Figure 6.2). This bringing together felt powerfully symbolic of a ritual of connection and completion. What was also happening simultaneously at this time was the fact that her stringing together of words was increasing, and instead of speaking in small disjointed phrases she was now beginning to make longer sentences. Each week towards the end of the session she would hold her painting up proudly and say 'there, finished'. Her expression was always joyful at these moments, and there was a strong sense of achievement and mastery. She would smile warmly and wrap her arms around herself, swaying slightly, whilst looking at her painting again before leaving the room.

Her death preceded her ability to finish all her paintings, but she had managed to complete a considerable number before she died. The work indicated to me that although this woman was clearly disabled by her cognitive deficits, a strong sense of renewal and rebirth had occurred during the course of the therapy. For me the image became 'shrine-like', and I wondered about the symbolic nature of the animals returning to the barn. The paintings appeared to be about night-time, and I thought about her ageing and the evening of her life. Her constant thanking me for having her suggested a mark of her pleasure at the experience of being there and creating the images. Her absorption with the image-making process appeared to leave the group behind and she seemed to be working at a deep level as if going somewhere else. Her quietness during the painting time also had a spiritual quality about its stillness and calmness.

Her paintings represented a fond and treasured memory that I felt she would take with her to the grave. The cradling and cuddling of herself when she completed a painting perhaps indicated the nourishment and joy she felt

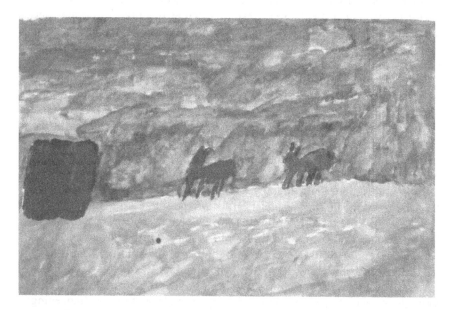

Figure 6.2

when recapturing these fond memories. Her need to get home to her mum who would have tea ready also gave me a sense of her returning to mother earth. Filling the gap in the paintings that occurred later in the therapy suggested many things to me. I thought about the process of filling in the gaps; sorting out unfinished business; tying up loose ends; repairing the split. There was a sense of completion as she filled the gaps in her previous paintings, and the meeting of the earth and the heavens felt very powerful.

Another woman was referred to art therapy because of her confusion about the recent death of her husband. Her family apparently felt it would be too upsetting for her to go his funeral and it was very clear she had not come to terms with his loss, behaving as if nothing had changed. She was 79 and there was an authoritative air about her presence. She was quite formal in greeting me, saying 'How do you do', and 'Pleased to meet you'. It was not clear how much she understood of what I was saying to her, but she was interested in the art materials on the table between us during the initial assessment session and she fingered them whilst attempting a verbal dialogue with me. My impression was that beneath the learnt social front her memory was significantly impaired, although she appeared to remember me when I collected her each week for the group.

At the beginning of her first art therapy group session she reached for a piece of white cartridge paper and then appeared to become stuck as if pondering what to do for a long time. Finally she noticed a potted plant on the window sill. 'Ah', she said, and went over to examine it more closely. She brought the plant back to the table and placed it in front of her. To the left of the paper she proceeded to paint the plant and plant pot and at the end of the session was very concerned about clearing up properly. Upon leaving the room after sessions she would often tell me that she had to go home to cook her husband's meal. This was a clear indication that she had not accepted his death, and I wondered how much she might be in denial.

Each week during her first series of sessions she went to the window and collected the same plant she had been painting before. She noticed her folder with her name on it, and I encouraged her to look inside as she struggled to find the opening. On discovering the painting inside she seemed pleased, but indicated that she could improve upon it.

This first image was very green and alive (see left-hand side of Figure 6.3), and after many weeks of painting it she moved her attention to the right-hand side of the paper. Without placing a plant pot in front of her for reference as before, she began painting another pot from her imagination. She worked more slowly and it took her the whole of this session to complete the outline. She returned to this painting over several weeks, and I was struck by the two rounded oblong shapes that were emerging (see right-hand side of Figure 6.3). Of note, after the sessions when she created this image she did not mention the need to cook a meal for her husband when she got home.

She talked more during the next session and was able to tell the group a

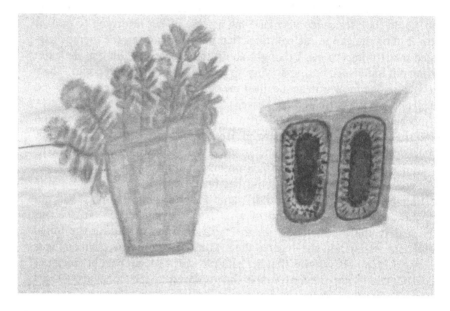

Figure 6.3

little about her past working life when she had been in a supervisory role. This sense of her being 'in charge' at work perhaps accounted for her formality and need to be in control, which I had witnessed in our sessions so far. Her talking more was encouraging, marking the development of trust being established in the therapy. In the movement from painting something in front of her on the left-hand side of the paper, to depicting something on the right from her imagination, the focus seemed to shift from an outer to an inner concern. I wondered what she was dealing with now at an unconscious level. In this session she concentrated on filling in the two rounded oblong areas with more brown paint. To me the image looked like two plots of earth. I began to think about death and cemeteries, and the fact that she had not visited the grave of her husband. She did not refer to her husband at the end of these sessions, and I wondered if through the image-making process she was resolving something about his death.

The following week she looked at her previous paintings for a while and then put them back in her folder and reached for a new piece of paper. She then seemed to be at a loss to know what to do with it. She first looked at me blankly, and then inspected the room, leaving her chair and walking around the table. Her interest settled on a pot of African violets on the window sill. She brought them to the table and spent most of the session painting the plant pot. Towards the end she then painted two African violets in blue paint to the left of the pot, and one single blue flower to the right. She painted in a few leaves, but left a space between the two flowers to the left and the single flower to the right. This made me think about pairing and separation, and her experience of being married and then widowed. At the end of this session she commented 'It's not finished' and then 'I'll have to finish it next time.' Symbolically this felt like a parallel connection between her image and the acknowledgement that something was unresolved in her life.

The weeks that followed seemed very much about an unconscious exploration of mortality. She would place the pot of African violets on the table in front of her and notice that some of the flowers had died, having become brown and dried up. She picked off the dead ones before continuing to paint. This picking off of the dead flowers felt a very powerful non-verbal acknowledgement of the bereavement she had suffered. She painted in brown around the edges of the pot and it felt as if she was reinforcing the container. She then settled to filling in the gap between the paired and single flowers by adding others in purple in between them. The original blue flowers still stood out (see Figure 6.4).

At the end of the group sessions she appeared preoccupied with making sure she cleared up properly. The clearing away in itself felt like a demonstration of the need to clear something up and sort something out in some way.

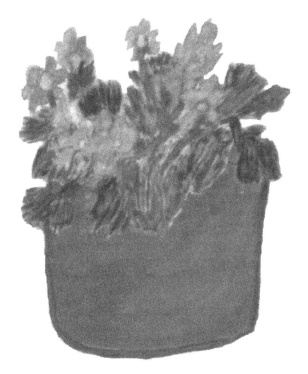

Figure 6.4

After one session I looked at her painting, which she had left out to dry, and turned it upside down out of interest. Upside down the painting looked to me like a gravestone with flowers at the base, much as one might expect to find in a cemetery (see Figure 6.5).

The following week she collected the plant from the window sill and again picked off the dead flowers, this time tending to the dead leaves as well. This was done in silence and felt like a mourning. I thought about my own visits to family graves and times when I had cleared away the dead flowers left there. She looked at the space to the right of the image, and then took the plant back to the window sill. She returned to the table and began a much darker painting, again from her imagination. What looked like another plant pot was created; it appeared to contain dead foliage (see right-hand side of Figure 6.6). Again, for me, images of cemeteries came up in my imagination as a response to her painting. At the end of this session she said: 'I'm on my own now, you know.' This was the first verbal acknowledgement of her situation, and felt very important in the therapy. She asked me: 'Do you know how old I am?' and then unsuccessfully struggled to tell me. 'I've forgotten', she said, and then 'I must be getting old', and she laughed. My sense was that she was really coming to terms with her situation now, and that the sessions

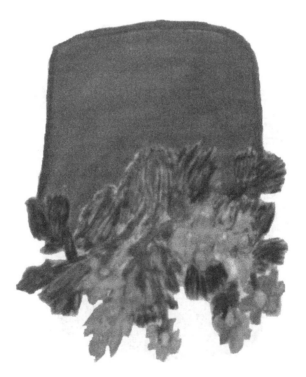

Figure 6.5

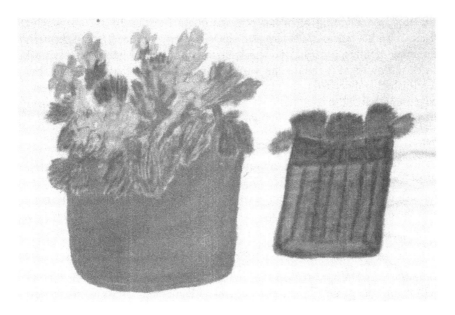

Figure 6.6

had demonstrated a significant change taking place. She continued with the previous painting, and again I was struck by how, if viewed upside down, it looked like a headstone. I felt something important had been laid to rest in the therapy and that words alone could not have facilitated this to happen.

Initially when she began to work in the group she appeared to be holding on to the past, both in her formal manner, that suggested her working years in a supervisory position, and in her desire to copy something rather than work from the imagination. Painting a plant in a pot also suggested a need in her to contain something rather than let it spill out, as did continually reinforcing the outline of the pots she painted. Clearing away at the end of sessions was also important to her, perhaps in order to keep things neat and under control, making sure there was no mess. These early ways of working seemed to allow the denial of her husband's death, and kept alive her belief that she was going home to cook his evening meal after our sessions.

Throughout the therapy there was a strong sense of life and death, pairing and separation in the imagery she created. The first painting appeared more green and lively; the later paintings were dulled in effect and seemed more lifeless. The paired and single blue flowers were to me powerfully symbolic of the break in her union with her husband. When she stopped mentioning going home to cook for her husband and adopted less formal language I sensed a greater letting go at a psychic level. She appeared to be involved in an unconscious exploration of mortality, and I believe the work she did in therapy was truly healing for her. I began to think about the ties that bind, and how by the letting go of her past she might free herself in some way in order to walk a new path. It was as if she was laying her dead to rest through the image-making process, and this was poignantly felt when she picked off the dead flowers of the plant she was painting. The sense that something was not finished and needed to be finished was very powerful. The verbal acknowledgement that she was on her own strongly suggested she had acknowledged her husband's death and was living in the here and now.

Having moved from a position of confusion and denial about her loss, to one of understanding and acceptance, proved that the therapy was transforming for her. It made me think about the many times I hear of people with a diagnosis of dementia not attending the funerals of their loved ones. It left me with questions. If older people with memory loss are denied involvement with the death of their loved ones, is it not surprising therefore that they find it more difficult to come to terms with the loss? Do such people need such protection from reality, particularly when they are struggling with reality anyway? These questions about the possible psychological harm that can come out of what appears, on the surface, to be a sensitive concern for the well-being and protection of the person with memory loss are interesting to me.

A 75-year-old man who was quite new to coming to the hospital was referred to me for individual art therapy because of his confusion about what was going on in his life. He was unable to express himself in a coherent manner verbally, and appeared very agitated about his situation. The staff felt that by having an opportunity to explore his feelings through the use of art materials he might become more settled within himself.

The initial meeting and first three sessions were very symbolic of his disorientation. He would be glad to meet me each time, although it was not clear whether he remembered who I was or why we were meeting. He seemed happy to walk with me to the therapy room, and each time, on the way there and the way back he would try to open the doors into other rooms. He walked in front of me quite often and pointed to notices and other signs around the hospital building. Once in the therapy room, he would not sit down, preferring to stand and walk about. Although this showed a restlessness in him, he did not appear to be agitated and seemed quite content to stay for about fifteen to twenty minutes each time. Then he would want to leave and beckon me to come with him. I tried to encourage him to stay longer, but he appeared strong in his conviction to leave. He managed the occasional word or two but did not seem able to string a sentence together.

In the following session he pointed more to things on the way and I again had the strong feeling he was taking charge and showing me round. Perhaps he felt he was a member of staff and I was a visitor, but it was difficult to know. When he investigated the art materials on the table I encouraged him to sit down, but he preferred to stand and move about as before.

Much of the next session was the same as the others except for the amount of time he spent rearranging the art materials, which was longer than before. He moved the paint pots, and lined up the crayons. It looked as if he was trying to organise things into distinct groups. He then separated the different types of materials, putting all the paints together in one place and all the pencils in another, and so on, until all the different materials were in uniform groups on the table. He then appeared to lose interest in this and wanted to leave early as usual. Every time he wanted to leave I would try to encourage him to stay longer, but with no success.

He always began the session by pacing around the room and looking into drawers and cupboards, and this led him to focus for a while on the table and the art materials. He would rearrange the art materials, and it appeared that by re-grouping them he was stimulating something within himself, seeming relieved afterwards. Because he had few words to say, it was impossible to know what was going on at an objective and conscious level. However, from a subjective viewpoint, the work seemed to be about taking charge in some way. It felt as if he was in control, particularly in the way he often went ahead of me as if to lead me, and also show me. I sensed the grouping of the art materials was an important process for him. I wondered how much this sorting out of the materials into groups might reflect a need within himself to organise and sort out his experience. Certainly, he did appear to be confused about what was going on. I never really knew how much he understood what I was saying to him and what we were doing, but I did feel there was a point to the work.

The need to be in control and in charge of the experience seemed important to him in these sessions. Although he did not engage with the art materials as I expected he might, the whole process of arranging them into distinct and same-type groups felt important. This may well have been symbolic of attempts to deal with his confusion.

I am left wondering about what value there may have been in his organising of the materials, and of the experience as a whole. Perhaps this was more about the denial of his disintegration and fragmentation. I sensed in his behaviour it was as if he was holding on to his perception of being in a useful and working role. If this was the case the work might have expressed a denial of retirement, or the redundancy associated with older age, especially when memory loss is apparent. Alternatively, if his experience of the world was as chaotic as I imagined it to be, the opportunity to organise and direct may have felt empowering in itself.

In art therapy the way materials are selected and manipulated, as well as any resulting artefacts and verbalisations that accompany the process, can provide clues as to what may be of concern to the individual. If people with memory loss experience difficulty in making themselves understood in the verbal mode, the art-making activity can provide an alternative non-verbal way of communication. The opportunity freely to create using art materials can be very healing and bring about a sense of achievement and control, and the opportunity of being better understood by others. In this way there is potential for the exploration of important thoughts, feelings and emotions, both conscious and unconscious, which may help to resolve hidden or inner conflicts.

A sense of continuity, privacy, familiarity and trust can be fostered by providing a consistent time and place, free of interruptions and distractions from outside. In a setting that encourages people to be themselves, free from external expectations, the person can become empowered. They can begin to organise their own experience and make their own choices through the use of art materials. This opportunity to be themselves and to be free to express and explore their feelings can be rare for older people.

Rooms offering quiet and privacy are often non-existent in places where older people who suffer memory loss spend time. In old people's homes, and hospital wards, it is not uncommon for people to have to share the rooms where they sleep. During the day it is also likely that the older person will be sitting in a large room with lots of other people. Potentially, in my view, a person's disorientation can increase the more distraction and disruption is happening around them. Sometimes people have mentioned their belief that they are in a waiting room when they are grouped together in a large day room full of chairs and activity. However, they are often unsure what it is they are waiting for and why they are there in the first place.

In the hospital setting I have often found it necessary to provide a space away from the area where the older person is usually situated. In order to make sure I can keep to a consistent time for therapy I begin and end the session where the person is staying in the hospital, be it a ward or day hospital setting. This means that a transition takes place whereby the person is escorted by me to and from the art therapy room. This type of beginning and ending raises a lot of interesting issues.

As therapy is voluntary it is important that the people I see feel they have a choice as to whether or not they wish to participate each week. Outpatients who are not suffering impaired memory will attend as they wish, without the therapist appearing on their doorstep every week as it were. By collecting the patients, the whole issue of older people in hospital care having choice and not being pushed into things against their wishes is brought sharply into focus. When I meet with the person I attempt to make sure that they know who I am, why I have come, and that what is being offered is optional. I respect their wishes if they do not want to come, and in this way they exercise their choice and make their own decisions.

Of course, the reality is that these people have special needs as they could not be expected to find their way to the art therapy room independently and would be likely to get lost if left to their own devices. I collect them myself because I do not feel it is appropriate to ask frequently overstretched nursing staff to escort them. As they are often over the age of 75, some of them are physically frail and may need or appreciate some reassurance and physical support. Therefore the issue of touch becomes an important one, and physical contact with this client group is common. Another observation about escorting the older person with memory loss is that the journey to and from the art therapy room evokes many comments about what they are leaving behind and going to. This can provide interesting insights into their own personal experience of attending hospital, and coming for therapy.

As mentioned earlier, initially upon arrival in the art therapy room it is often clear from a range of comments, facial expressions and body language that both the environment and what takes place within it are unfamiliar. Given time, memories associated with the venue develop and gradually empower the individual as he or she begins to indicate a sense of knowing and belonging. Where to hang their coats and hats becomes familiar without being shown or reminded. They get used to where to sit and often occupy the same positions as if they have their own particular place in the room. A knowing through experience takes place as they learn where to get the art materials and where their previous work is kept if they want to review it or continue working on a past piece. Therefore they are able to act independently of me to a considerable extent and take some control over their lives. The process of becoming familiar with the people and the environment can be slow, but providing there is consistency their memories from one week to the next can be seen to gain in capacity. As each individual organises their own experience in the room there is often a strong sense of re-integration apparent, where perhaps a perceived general lack of ability or control appears to be rediscovered.

In the art therapy group consistency of membership is important. The faces become familiar, and even though the people in the group do not always know their own names, let alone the names of other members, the faces can be recognised. Absences are noticed, and if someone leaves the group abruptly, perhaps due to moving into a nursing home or through death, the issue of mortality becomes poignant for us all.

In preparing to die I believe that many older adults would welcome the opportunity to work through the various experiences of their lives with another in therapy, and perhaps by so doing tie up some loose ends. This type of internal stock-take and opportunity to explore unresolved conflicts and suppressed feelings can be very liberating. Giving expression to the belief system in terms of what the person believes might happen after their death, both to themselves and those they might be leaving behind, also seems an important area to be addressing at this time in one's life.

Chapter 7

Real world or fantasy?

Ken Evans

From the moment that someone is 'diagnosed' as 'having dementia', to their eventual 'placement' in a 'care home', the processes involve a variety of social agents whose understanding of the condition is partial and confused.

Some of the reasons for this confusion are a consequence of different perspectives of the main agencies, the Health Services, Social Services, and the independent providers of care. At a different level of analysis this confusion reflects a particular ideology communicated through political, economic and social policies concerning mental health issues. Other reasons are more the result of a general culture of confusion about mental illness, which is disseminated through public attitudes and values.

For anyone who enters this bizarre world – for that is what it is – becomes helplessly entrapped in a series of processes which systematically degrade their independence, individuality and personhood. Each part of the sequence of this process, while appearing to be cohesive and continuous, is in fact isolated, each agency defending its own territory, with error being amplified at each stage. Generally the first point of contact for the individual – patient, client, sufferer: define them however we may – is the GP, their own doctor, who in the majority of cases has limited knowledge and understanding of dementia.

In a small sample (15) of local GPs who were interviewed for the purposes of this chapter, none had any clear knowledge of how to assess patients for dementia, or an understanding of the various types of dementia. One GP admitted that when he did his training very little was known about dementia, and consequently sufferers were considered to be 'hopeless cases'.

Social workers, mainly care managers working for local authorities are slightly better informed, for they are the go-betweens, the 'brokers' who manage a client's transition from 'home life' to 'care home'. Some will have detailed information about the condition, and will have constructed their own personal view of dementia, but will also assume that GPs have competently diagnosed patients. At this point in the process, the patient becomes the client, and will be assessed according to the local authority's assessment procedures. These procedures vary between local authorities, but are based on some version of a 'risk matrix'. This assessment is carried out by whoever is available in the Social Services locality team, experienced or otherwise, and is intended to measure levels of need for care, priorities which eventually relate to so-called 'care packages'. In ordinary language this means what is going to happen to the 'client', where they are going to go, and how much it is going to cost.

Referral to Social Services is the point of no return, for this is the focal point at which 'reality' concerning dementia sufferers is constructed. This, without realising it, was also the point at which I entered the fantasy world of dementia care. After teaching academic psychology for a few years, and drifting into medical and social work training, I was approached by a large county council social work department to conduct a research project looking at the interface between 'social' and 'health'. The principal concern was to research problems associated with 'hospital discharges'. Thus I had free access to hospital trusts, hospital departments, occupational therapists, general practices, psychiatric departments, special hospitals, directors of social services, senior managers, care staff, care home managers – in fact the whole caboodle. When I started the project I was unaware that at least two other previous attempts to 'crack the problems of hospital discharge' had occurred, with data, results, and reports, etc. simply disappearing. My learning curve involved interviewing key operators in the systems, travelling many miles between agencies and, bit by bit, building up a picture of how one public agency failed to connect with other public agencies. To anyone with a curious mind and a researcher's interest, it was both fascinating and appalling to observe the extent and levels of institutional incompetence. Each of the agencies inhabited its own small world, while operating with all the confidence as if it governed the universe. Their peculiar language, policies and procedures embodied a kind of code which only its own operators understood, and which required a kind of allegiance from its troops. As a consultant researcher, and therefore 'an outsider' without any particular axe to grind, I held an almost anonymous status. The various troops diligently provided the vital information I requested, and also unburdened their souls to me. Some of them used the interviews as a means of venting their own frustrations, others contributed to their own disappointment by believing that what they told me would eventually lead to some sane way of working, some magical master plan. Although I was able to maintain separateness from the machinery of care, I had acquired an identity, which provided a means of contact with all the major players in the system, and a unique vantage point from which to observe the system.

After a brief spell back teaching, I was recruited by a large care company, specialising in the provision of nursing and social care for dementia sufferers. With my working knowledge of how the statutory agencies functioned I was viewed as an 'expert', and among other things was expected to provide a sort of protection for the company against local authority criticism. The relationship between the independent providers of 'care' and the 'purchasers' – local authority social services departments – is a pernicious one. Very few local authorities have the capacity themselves to provide services for dementia sufferers; care in one form or another is purchased from 'independent providers' at the lowest price possible. The providers, which include anything from a purpose-built home with trained staff to a converted old domestic dwelling with untrained and low-paid staff, supply services of variable quality, at a price that allows some profit. I had visited several whilst working on the research project, and had learned from various sources of the different reputations, of cases of abuse and neglect. The company I worked for served four counties and had several homes, and because at some point in time needs had outstripped supply some of their homes had been registered for maximum capacity.

My main role was to review care procedures and introduce a training programme to meet new local authority demands. But as the training costs exceeded the tiny budget for this purpose I became a kind of negotiator between the company and the various Social Services departments, filling the beds as they became vacant and agreeing a price. After a very short period of time my value to the company was measured in terms of profit, which was measured in terms of the number of beds occupied. In the marketplace of care, price was the most significant determinant of making a placement, and that marketplace included competitors willing to cut the price to fill their beds. Profit margins were based on a 90 per cent plus capacity, and when there was a death or a fall the atmosphere of the entire home changed. The home owners and the managers reminded everyone of the need to make savings, and dropped hints of possible cut-backs, the catering manager being told to reduce spending, the home manager to cut overtime. And I would be asked to ring round to the local authority's Social Services departments and trawl for more clients. But this only occurred occasionally, because usually there was an uninterrupted flow of residents, filling the vacant spaces of those who had recently departed this world, the only means of escape from this end-of-the-road place. Sometimes whilst driving home after work, thoughts about what was happening, and about how residents came and sometimes died after a very short time, reminded me of other situations where people queued, and took their turn to die. To those who worked in the various agencies who participated in this process, each seemed to regard their part as a positive benefit, each contributing to the solution of a health or social problem. Dementia became a kind of slogan, the name of an enemy, an impossible disease, a death sentence.

The route to the care home usually begins with an individual's partner or friend contacting the GP's surgery asking for advice, their loved one exhibiting unusual behaviour, such as wandering, forgetfulness, aggressiveness, sexual disinhibition. Some doctors immediately refer the patient to Social Services, many willing to diagnose a condition they know almost nothing about. Others would refer patients to specialist gerontology services in local hospitals. In the care homes I visited I had access to medical records. The doctors' notes were mostly too vague in the descriptions of the indicators and symptoms they considered to define dementia. There were sometimes references to Alzheimer's, or other forms of dementia, without any evidence of any tests being carried out, and possibly without understanding that for some types of dementia the only definite identification is by autopsy! My guess is that doctors do not like to admit to their ignorance, but wish to solve problems. Social workers' assessments do not assess the symptoms, their assessment is an attempt to assess care needs, and frequently they take the doctor's diagnosis as 'factual' and valid. Their concern always includes the client's partner, husband or wife, and sometimes their needs take precedence over the sufferer's needs. If, for example, the spouse is being abused, or is unable to deal with the problems of a 'dementing' partner, then the most frequent solution is to remove the client into a care home. Thus the saga begins, for in that process there are all the problems relating to the quality of care that might be provided, funding issues, along with the location of a suitable home and problems with travelling and visits – plus, of course, the guilt engendered by the part played by the partner in their loved one's incarceration.

When small care homes are contacted by care managers, if there is a vacancy, the owner/manager bases their decision whether to accept the client on their own criteria, usually price or level of dependence of the client. I have heard descriptions such as 'He's a nice quiet elderly gentleman, . . . no trouble, . . . etc.', or 'elderly and confused, should fit in very nicely, etc.'. When one of the company homes had to be closed for financial reasons, and the residents were distributed to a number of smaller homes, I was able to visit the homes and gauge the services on offer, and discovered an amazing world of small-homes culture. In any given area the homes' staff all know each other, sometimes moving between homes for an increase in pay, and consequently sharing inside information. Almost every feature of home-life is compared, and biographical details of residents described in terms of a cinematic narrative. For the larger homes, Social Services care managers expect a formal assessment, which might be carried out by a qualified RMN, or in the case of larger companies by a qualified psychologist.

When 'assessment' was added to my other duties I realised that I had lost my neutral status and had been drawn deeply into the unreal world of dementia care. With an academic background in both psychology and sociology I suddenly found myself searching for a paradigm or model which might at least provide some sense of direction. I had already observed enough to know that the field of dementia care, and perhaps the whole field of mental health care, was unreal, a closed self-defining system, and perhaps not about care at all but about containment and control. Also I had spoken to enough people to know that assessment was frequently the means to an end, an essential rite of passage which would somehow justify all future decisions concerning an individual. I was already aware of various assessment procedures and documents, such as the Mini-Mental State Examination (MMSE), and Reality Orientation Assessment Lists, but soon acquired other sets of assessment documents from other 'dementia professionals'. These included a Neuropsychiatric Inventory (NPI) intended to screen for 'delusions, hallucinations, agitation, aggression, depression, dysphoria, anxiety, euphoria, apathy, disinhibition, and aberrant motor behaviour'; the Health of the Nation Outcome Scales (HoNOS); the Behavioral Pathology in Alzheimer's Disease Rating Scale (BEHAVE!! AD); the Functional Assessment Staging (FAST); and the Cohen–Mansfield Agitation Inventory (CMAI), to name a few! I also visited a 'memory clinic' attached to a large provincial hospital for further guidance about how I might approach assessing people who had already been labelled as 'dementing'.

Such is the culture of confusion in Social Services and NHS hospitals concerning mental health issues, that anyone armed with a full magazine of 'assessment procedures' is welcomed as a 'new gun'. Part of the reason for this is the lack of cohesiveness of mental health perspectives between the several agencies concerned with the provision of care. So the 'new gun' will be seen as someone who can solve some of their problems. But there are other institutional pressures that are a direct consequence of central government policies, especially those policies which claim to be 'effective', 'efficient' and 'value for money related'. These are translated into league tables and have become part of the system. Each part of the system, with its own culture and traditions, is under pressure to maximise patient 'throughput', a magical term that is central to the *modus operandi* of the entire present system. To begin with, general practices cannot deal with dementia cases; the pressure for them is to make a fast referral – in other words, to pass them down the line. In cases where dementia sufferers are hospitalised for other injuries or conditions, there is pressure to limit their stay to the minimum time possible; that is, to 'unblock' beds. Blocked beds have an impact throughout hospital departments, for where funding is related to efficiency, as a consequence resources, and even staff careers, can suffer. But vulnerable dementia patients cannot easily be discharged back into their own homes, and the pressure is passed further down the line to the local Social Services departments. From this point onwards the dementia sufferer/client becomes totally defenceless.

Finally the 'pressures' to solve or deal with one of society's problems, the containment of someone who might be confused, agitated, or threatening in some way, came to rest with me. Almost without noticing I had become part of that mad world. Requests for me to carry out assessments came from all directions: from GPs, hospital ward managers, Social Services care managers, local authority housing departments, managers of care and nursing homes, and sometimes from an individual's family. Despite my guarded feeling of discomfort I arrived at a care home to conduct my first 'assessment'. I had already decided to loosely apply some of the categories used in the MMSE

(Mini-Mental State Examination), concentrating on the person's insight of who they are and where they are. I also hoped that I would be able to get a brief idea of family history from the care home manager, and that I could build an assessment around this information. My reception had been lubricated by communications between the home and the network of 'professionals', Social Services care managers, etc.: I was told that the client I was to assess had outgrown her present placement. It was a small home, lost somewhere in the country, run by a family, with care staff more like extended family members, and Betty (not her real name), the client, had started to become 'difficult'. After more than three years of 'good behaviour' she had started to become unco-operative and incontinent. At this stage I was unaware of any hidden agenda about how care homes select their clients, and then unload them on to others when they require 'more care' than the funding body are prepared to pay. Betty, I was informed, had now 'deteriorated', had become 'argumentative' and needed specialised care. The home's manager hoped that I would be able to assess this deterioration and be able to arrange a transfer for Betty to a more suitable home.

The assessment interview lasted about half an hour. She had been told that someone was coming to see her, but no reasons had been given for my visit, and not surprisingly she was confused by this. She was frail and clearly took pride in her appearance. For the first few minutes we chatted about her hair, and a 'perm' she had recently had. There was also a child-like quality in her acceptance of my questions. Although she was not sure what day or month it was, she knew she had been in the home for a long time. She introduced me to a small toy bear wearing a hand-made military tunic. He looked like a soldier and had the same name as her deceased husband, who I later learned had been a much-decorated 'hero' in the parachute regiment during the Second World War. From my questions it was clear that she was unaware that she had been either unco-operative or argumentative, and mentioned more than once that she was happy where she was. I took this to mean that she might have guessed that there were plans to move her, in which case she indicated remarkable insight, because she would need to apply the very small cues from my visit. I later discussed my impressions of Betty with her Social Services care manager, who was adamant that she had to be moved because of her deterioration, and requested a written report of the assessment. She required a formal statement based on a recognised scored test. It was impossible to form any valid impression of Betty's care needs from her medical notes, or from the brief anecdotal records held by the care home, and I considered a half-hour interview as inadequate to make any reasonable judgement. Finally I agreed to write a brief statement, after which the wheels were set in motion and Betty turned up in one of the company homes.

Gradually I learned the range of expectations of my new role from the key players, which always excluded any direct input from the clients themselves. Sometimes all I could do was to apply my own ethical considerations, and produce a report that would redirect clients in other directions. I had been told briefly that Mr Grey had been awaiting discharge from the hospital for several months, and that he had been admitted after setting fire to his flat, where he had lived by himself for several years. I had nothing else to go by other than the half-hour conversation with him. He was nearly 60 and had the battered appearance of someone who had a 'drinking habit', as he was able to confirm, but was now obviously 'dried-out' and spruced up for the interview. During the conversation he came across as remarkably insightful, and managed to highlight incidents in his life that accounted for his isolated lifestyle. He spoke with sadness and disappointment at the breakup of his marriage, the involvement of a close friend in the affair, and the kindness of a woman in renting him his flat. He also powerfully expressed his sense of timelessness and desolation in the hospital, and his eagerness to escape. He clearly saw me as someone who could assist him in this. Most of the questions I asked were intended to reveal indications of dementia: short-term memory, attention, orientation, activity disturbances, etc. As far as I could tell he was fine. Near the end of the interview I asked him what kind of accommodation he preferred, and he suggested a room or flat, near a town and some allotments where he could grow things; he obviously did not expect to go into a care home. Finally I put it to him that living on his own might lead to him repeating the incident that had led him there: setting fire to his home. Then I asked him why he had started the fire. Up to this point the conversation had been relaxed and rational and conventional, but now he explained how bugs had invaded his kitchen from underneath the skirting board, battalions of them, and especially when he was cooking his bacon sandwiches. I suggested that to start a fire as a means of dealing with the bugs was dangerous, and that it might have been simpler to use an insecticide powder or something similar. He simply said that there were too many of them, and that only fire would do the trick, and besides they only came when he cooked bacon, and they came to laugh at him. When I asked why they should laugh at him, he simply shrugged his shoulders. I referred to Mr Grey's 'delusion behaviour' in the assessment report only briefly, and suggested to his care manager that a short period in a care home would provide a more relaxed atmosphere during which Mr Grey could be monitored for ability to live independently. During the four months that Mr Grey was living in one of the homes I frequently visited, I had several brief conversations with him. On each occasion he told me that he thought most of the other residents were crazy, and that he might 'catch it' if he stayed there too long. It occurred to me that he was probably right about this, for his surroundings and contacts would be sufficient to drive anyone crazy. He finally moved to a warden-controlled flat, and made many friends, successfully living independently.

After more than a year of assessing dementia sufferers I had gained enough experience to assess the wider social circumstances which placed individuals in the system. In cases where individuals were married, partners would seek help in dealing with 'unusual' behaviour. Sometimes this would be progressive forgetfulness. For example, one case involved a man who would frequently return home after taking his dog for a walk, but without the dog. He would either leave it tied up somewhere or have given it away. In another case a woman complained that her husband had become over-amorous, and would follow her around their house trying to engage her sexually. In most of the 'sexually disinhibited' cases, I came to suspect that the social workers' descriptions of the 'sexual attacks' were influenced by their own personal attitudes towards sexual matters, and their own sexuality.

Partners and family carers are sometimes identified by care managers as the main reason for admission of a dementia sufferer to a care home. On the one hand the partner wants their spouse to receive proper care, while on the other they wrestle with their feelings of guilt for having colluded in their partner's incarceration. The dynamics of conjugal relationships are always complex, and it is almost impossible to unravel the tangled web of emotions and memories that lead to a cry for help. But once the process is set in motion there is no stopping it, and there is an inevitability about its progress and outcome.

Assessment in mental health has several definitions. In psychological terms it is an attempt to measure atypical behaviour of individuals. As such it is part of a 'medical model' and presumes that there are categories of behaviour that can be identified as abnormal or atypical, which can be used to define someone as ill. For social workers, assessment concerns 'needs' and 'risks', not only of an individual but also of others – sometimes close relatives, sometimes wider society. These usually are based on a risk-matrix table that requires ticks in little boxes. If it became common knowledge that individuals could be incarcerated in what Erving Goffman has described as 'total institutions' on the strength of a few ticks in boxes, or on the whim of a psychologist, there would be general public unease.

The present system of mental health care, which includes dementia care, is self-sustaining and self-validating; it has only two components, patients and operatives, one group defining reality for the other. The distinguishing process that separates the two groups is assessment, and assessment is the 'official' measurement of madness. Assessment tools, the various lists of questions, represent an outsider's view of an insider's subjective state of mind, and is derived from the canons of psychology, with its focus on the individual or, more correctly, certain aspects of an individual. There can be no reasonable objection to the idea of assessment in itself, but, like so many other attempts to apply psychological concepts in real situations, these concepts and processes becomes reified. And this reification occurs within a particular social and political framework, a framework that increasingly depends on measurement. All assessment tests currently used incorporate a scoring system and have as much validity as IQ tests. Furthermore, it is clear that assessment methods necessarily are consistent with the rest of the system and framework of mental health care. But the assessment test is arguably the most pernicious part of the system, because it is the point at which a person is separated from the real world and enters the unreal world of dementia care. This is also the point of no return, for included in the description 'dementia' is the knowledge that there is no cure, a modern kind of leprosy which demands separation from the real world, and from one's closest family and friends. But if the present methods of assessment are unsatisfactory then so is the whole system. It would be pointless to change the focus of assessment, which concentrates on the disabling mental and physical conditions of an individual and humanising it, without changing the rest of the system. Raising questions about the nature of assessment might be one way of challenging the whole current system and the thinking which underlies and justifies it.

The categories we use to think with are culturally bound, and we all invest large measures of belief in what we understand as our way of life and how it reflects reality. For most of us most of the time there is very little opportunity or need to discuss our lives in this way, for we are too busy getting through our days. But occasionally an idea comes along which challenges a common assumption, and perhaps gains credibility, even the idea of reality itself. Mental illness is part of that reality, and our common assumptions about it are challenged in an everyday sense and through the ideas of philosophy, anthropology, literature, etc. The ideas of Thomas Szasz, R.D. Laing, Michel Foucault, Roy Porter, and others have trickled through the system, and have sometimes flowed out the other side with little effect. But the grains of doubt they leave behind remain as a constant irritant, reminding the operatives of the system that something might be wrong with their practice. The overwhelming power of institutions limits our ability to influence change, but as Kuhn's theory of scientific revolutions suggests, internal stresses in any system eventually lead to 'paradigmatic shifts' – not small adjustments that continue to make the system run, but compete mind shifts that change the ways that people think and feel about things, producing new explanations and new ways of working. It is my view that modern society is like a tightrope walker teetering on the cusp of a new world-view, about society in general and life in particular. Part of that revolution will concentrate on the social conditions, which account for illness, and will shift our concentration from a 'chemical-based' approach to an appreciation of other approaches. These will include recognition of alternative explanations, and the richness of a multicultural approach where social values are concentrated on personal relationships.

All current assessment inventories for the assessment of dementia-type illnesses include sections which purport to measure 'personal insight' and 'orientation'. In other words, these are attempts to assess whether an individual knows who and where they are. But the circumstances and the manner in which the assessment is carried out can add to the confusion experienced by the individual, especially as the questions and the context in which they are asked are unlikely to relate to the individual's life experience. A phenomenological approach to assessment would take into account individuals' lifestyles and social experience, and would also employ sensitive methods and techniques relative to the individual being assessed. This is something we should all work towards if the rhetoric in documents emphasising 'patient choice' is to become reality.

Chapter 8

Living with dementia
Interview with Neil McArthur

Diane Waller

Neil McArthur is the co-ordinator of the Brighton and Hove branch of the Alzheimer's Society. This is a very progressive branch, thanks to Neil and his team, and our conversation reveals something about Neil's determination to bring about change, and my own struggle to understand a bit more about the meaning of dementia. The Alzheimer's Society is a registered charity, which has obtained Approved Provider status from Brighton and Hove Council.

D: Neil, how did you get involved in working with people with dementia?

N: My last job was as an academic registrar at a university. I took early retirement, and after spending some time thinking what to do, what I thought was a purely administrative job with the Alzheimer's Society came up. The reason I chose this job was that my grandmother had dementia and I remember the turmoil that she was in and the problems my parents experienced through her dementia. I thought perhaps I could use some of that experience to have an input into the job at the Society. I thought it was purely administrative, though, and had I known what it would turn out to be I probably wouldn't have applied for it!

D: So how long have you been doing this now, Neil?

N: Fourteen years, always in the Brighton branch.

D: When you first took on the job, how did you find it?

N: I found that a lot of professionals were as ignorant about dementia as I was, which was quite surprising. I also found that carers were very unsupported, that facilities that were offering care for people with dementia were ill-informed about the illness and about its impact on carers and family members.

D: The diagnosis of dementia can often be quite terrifying, can't it, for the person who receives it and their immediate family?

N: I think it is one of the worst diagnoses that people can receive, because of the negativity around the words 'Alzheimer's' and 'dementia', the thought of the lack of the positivities that the person will have. Plus there's always that thought that if my parent, my wife has it, partner has it, does that mean my children will have it, or I might get it. So there's the fear of inherited illness. And there's also the fear that GPs have around dementia: they don't want to give bad news, they are reluctant to make such a clear statement to people they have been GP to, and perhaps become a friend to, over a period of time.

D: I think that 14 years ago the term 'Alzheimer's' wasn't really understood by many people, except something to be frightened about. I remember seeing someone at an airport, being helped by a relative, and people around saying he must have Alzheimer's. I thought it would be the worst thing ever to happen.

N: People were always asking, what's the difference between senile dementia, dementia and Alzheimer's. It was thought they were three different illnesses. People thought Alzheimer's was a form of insanity, and in fact GPs very rarely gave the diagnosis because their diagnostic skills in this area were not all that sound. People were told they had dementia which might be of the Alzheimer's type. They were not invited to have scans which might have given a clearer diagnosis.

D: So what would have happened to somebody in that state 14 years ago?

N: The comment that patients and carers would have had in those days is that it is going to get difficult and you had better prepare yourself for the future. No more than that, and certainly a strong indication that things wouldn't get better. The thrust would be, have you considered residential care?

D: . . . that would be going almost immediately to the idea of getting put away . . .

N: Care really didn't come into it, it was more about control.

D: The idea of going away and getting rid of the problem . . .

N: Yes, people wouldn't have thought about therapies, maybe a day centre, but it would be a day centre where you were fed and taken home. Day care then was more like 10 o'clock to 3 o'clock, and though as a carer you were encouraged to have one or two weeks' break there weren't facilities to allow you to take advantage of that. Let alone was there any appreciation of the impact that knowing that the person you are caring for has a dementia, and the support that you as carer would need. From the outside, it seemed obvious that if you were given that sort of news about a relative, the impact on you could be as great, if not greater, than on the person with dementia. Quite often the person with dementia was in the moderate to severe stage when the diagnosis was given, therefore perhaps knowing they had a dementia might not have meant a great deal to them. But to the family, it would have. The person and their family would be sent away, perhaps to contact our Society.

D: So when you started work with the Society here, what was the set up?

N: We had a bedroom converted to an office that the Social Services gave us in one of their residential care homes. We weren't accessible to the public. We ran a very small relief care scheme, five relief carers visited about twenty people. Now we have fourteen relief carers going to about ninety people per week, two carers in the day centre for younger people with dementia, monthly newsletter, mini holidays for carers, carers' awareness training, dementia awareness training for residential care workers. So that shows how we have grown. We are now recognised as partners by the statutory services and we have more respect from those services for the work we do, which is an enormous step forward. Although it can be a bit frightening because we are often seen as 'the experts', but none of us are formally trained. It's all done through our experience and personal research and talking to people.

D: That development hasn't been achieved without a struggle.

N: It has been hard getting funding. We still lurch from uncertainty to uncertainty. We provide a service which the statutory services can't provide, without which a lot of people would have to go into residential care.

D: In a city like Brighton and Hove, with the elderly population, it is an enormous problem which couldn't begin to be faced by the statutory services.

N: East and West Sussex have the largest population of people with dementia of any county. It's a huge catchment area, and a growing problem. There are only one or two centres of excellence.

D: I have the impression that as far as medicine is concerned it hasn't been a popular area of specialisation?

N: It might be better now there is Aricept, the anti-dementia drug, and a more positive approach – living with dementia rather than dying with dementia, and I think that has aroused people's enthusiasm. The Alzheimer's Society should take some credit for that because we have shown that by using initiative and being bold about some of the work, people with dementia can still have a quality of life. It's not just in receiving, but they can give a great deal back.

D: I suppose it is getting away from the idea that once someone has dementia, that is it . . . might as well give up, and everybody gives up . . . a culture of negativity and despair. To change that culture is quite a task, in terms of training presumably . . .

N: As far as training is concerned, it is about changing attitudes: both of care workers and managers. Which ones do you start with first? Well I've tried to attack both! Without the managers on board, care workers can come up with ideas, but if managers don't sign up to them, then the care workers get frustrated. Without actually showing to care workers, yes you can achieve something, then they won't trust managers who come up with ideas they think are too idealistic . . . so it is a two-pronged attack. As a local branch we offer training both to managers and to care workers.

D: Can you describe to me a typical training session for managers and for care workers?

N: For care workers, we would be offering three main sessions, one would be on the difference between dementia and other illnesses, the second about communication and how to tackle what we perceive as challenging behaviour, then the third session would be around a person-centred care approach. So we are starting to care for the person not the illness. For managers it would be very similar. We need to put across these ideas because you have a lot of staff in residential care who have no training, no knowledge of dementia. In theory I could start up a residential care home, with no experience of hands-on care! There is only one privately registered nursing home in the whole of Brighton . . . and ten residential care homes . . . so we really are struggling.

D: You mean people could go somewhere where there was no understanding whatsoever about dementia?

N: Yes. Certainly. Some people who have a milder form of dementia can receive good quality of care, but my personal fear is that because of the lack of decent places people stay at home longer and we are starting to expect carers to take on roles of unpaid staff.

D: That could put a very big burden on carers.

N: To add on to the guilt they already have about not being able to cope . . .

D: If you had to tell someone that their partner had dementia, how would you go about it?

N: It is knowing the person, and the relationships they have, but I think I would start by asking the carer what their perceptions of dementia were. You do need to be honest, but it would depend if you used the word 'Alzheimer's', or talked about severe memory loss; and I think you should be honest. The question you will be asked is, how long until they get worse . . . or die . . . you have to say that it is progressive. You have to say that you just don't know how long till it gets worse . . . or how long the person will live.

D: I think I read that it is usually about seven years for Alzheimer's . . .

N: Quite often there is a big gap between the first signs of Alzheimer's, and at that point people with dementia and their carers often try to deny it, or disguise it, so it is possibly three or four years before they seek help and get a diagnosis . . . often when I speak to a family they may say they noticed something two years ago, and on investigating you find out it was more than that. But who can blame them not wanting to do anything then? It's only now that there's some hope . . .

D: Yes, it could be that they noticed a certain absent-mindedness, or a withdrawal, or retirement from the world. Which makes me think about retirement from work and its effects . . . I think it is a very interesting question about the crisis of identity and depression which occurs sometimes when people retire, when they retire from a job where they have had an important role. Then they have no work and sometimes they feel they have no alternatives. They have all sorts of fantasies about travelling around etc., having a wonderful time . . . but they have lost their identity to a large extent. In my experience that seems to happen to men more than women . . . I wonder if there could be any connection . . .

N: I am sure that could bring about depression, but dementia is organic . . .

D: But I find it fascinating how much organic problems are exacerbated by psychological factors and how much psychological problems could bring about organic problems. It is a really difficult one . . . which I was always struggling with during Dan's illness . . .

N: Because we are saying that dementia attacks the cells, which gives you your identity, then your personality is affected, you will be changed. It sounds odd to say this, but some people seem to 'take to' dementia smoothly, and others seem to be frightened, so what is making that difference?

D: A colleague's husband had severe Parkinson's, and with the large doses of L-dopa he took as the illness got worse, he developed a psychosis. She said that because he had been a rather quiet, passive sort of person who liked to stay in, in a way the movement problems of Parkinson's didn't seem to be that much of a problem. He wasn't an active, athletic type, but later on he manifested his problems in night-time wanderings, which she found very difficult. He seemed not to experience anger or frustration that much, but she experienced it for him and was quite overwhelmed.

N: That's why it is very difficult when family members ask us, what is the future, because you really can't tell. The common core is that it will get worse, but how people react you can't tell. Some get more extrovert, angry, use language that we never thought they could, others don't seem much affected. I wouldn't say my grandmother aged a great deal in terms of physical appearance, but there are others who physically age rapidly, take on the appearance of an old person very quickly.

D: It seems that the physical problems attached to dementia are very severe . . .

N: But sometimes it seems that the dementia staves off the physical problems attached to old age, though . . .

D: What about distressing things like incontinence . . .

N: There is a difference between incontinence and toileting problems. Incontinence to me is a physical disability not being able to control bladder and bowels. Dementia is a lack of knowing where or when you should go. It's to do with social conditioning, which bit by bit goes. Some people get over that and realise where they are, where is appropriate to go to the toilet and they keep that memory. Some people with dementia feel moistness in their clothes, they recognise the discomfort of being wet, but others appear not to notice.

D: So they have forgotten the routine . . . and maybe blanked out the result through shame?

N: When we are babies we go anywhere but then we are taught when and where to go . . . dementia strips our memory of the sensation of needing to go to the toilet, takes away the feeling . . . all this about understanding the voice of dementia, we can only do it to some degree . . . can't really know . . .

D: The person themselves seems to be in a world which is totally undifferentiated, with sensation and perception all muddled up.

N: I recall that my own grandmother was doubly incontinent and became very aggressive and gave us no clues, no body language to us as to what she was feeling.

D: How did your parents react to that?

N: Even now my parents say, why are you doing this work? They can't connect with that time. I think that is based on their own sense of failure. Even now, my mother will say, did we do the right thing? Could we have done better?

D: Do you find that is a common feeling among carers?

N: I think it is. Our branch prides itself on supporting carers, till well after their relative goes into residential care. When an ex-carer is talking to a current carer, you still see those doubts. You can't see the illness, you can only see the effects of the illness. You can't blame the person because they are not there. So you blame yourself. It is always: I should have done this, or if I hadn't have done that . . . there is a sense of anger that nobody tells you what to expect. My mother had to cope with my grandmother's illness (her mother-in-law) and felt that she wasn't prepared. She had no support for caring for my grandmother on her own, who got to the stage where she was not only incontinent but quite violent, so she had to make the decision for her to go into residential care.

D: That is a very hard thing to do. I imagine she had no alternative then. You have mentioned Aricept, I suppose it is the first medication that gives some hope. Have you seen any effects on the persons you come into contact with?

N: Aricept. It has to be put into context. It isn't a cure, but it gives some hope. When it first came on to the market, carers would phone us up saying, how can we get hold of it? They were prepared to sell everything to get it. There are persons on our books who have been on it for five years and the carers would say that they have seen improvements. Because we didn't know the people prior to their taking the drug, it is difficult for us to say. It seems to be prescribed more readily now, because at first this health authority was very reluctant to prescribe it. There are a lot of ethical problems around the use of Aricept but there have been changes noted, and also some severe rejections. It has to be explained to people with dementia and carers that there is no guarantee there will be a good outcome and it could be a bad one.

D: So if somebody had, say, fairly mild dementia, it might be prescribed, and they could be on it for about five years.

N: It only works on some people with dementia, and they have to be regularly assessed. If the person's ability didn't change, then the drug would have worked its course. If their scores on the psychometric tests had deteriorated then they would be put back on it.

D: Is it expensive?

N: I don't think so, about £1,000 a year. Compare that to the cocktail of drugs which cancer sufferers have to take . . . But if you multiply this by all the people with dementia, and the fact that it isn't a cure, it only works on some people, you can see that some health authorities might be hesitant. But £1,000 a year only equates to three weeks' residential care! It is a stepping stone, at least you have got a foundation, a step forward. The people on it are guinea pigs for the future. It could be an advancement.

D: It is a bit like when L-Dopa (dopamine) for Parkinson's came in. That was rather hit and miss at first . . .

N: What it has done is make people think, if we are trying to hold this illness at a moderate level, we now have to think about the quality of life that we give to dementia sufferers. So I think it has made a difference to the philosophy of care. The person with dementia is able to say, for a longer period of time, I don't like what is happening to me, do something about it. This has been very obvious at our day centre for younger people, where several people are on the drug.

D: I'd like you to say something about how you feel about the new centre . . .

N: A long journey, personal crusade. We had been asked earlier on in the Society about younger people. Carers would phone up in desperation, but we could do very little. We weren't sure about how many people there were and there seemed to be a reluctance on behalf of the statutory services to find out. We managed to raise some money and did some research. We found 100 people in Brighton and Hove and Lewes with early onset dementia, and we were able to ask them, and their carers, what they needed. A clear message came through – a simpler diagnostic route and appropriate day-care facilities. The diagnostic route I felt was better met by the South Downs Health Trust, but the day centre facility I felt we could do something about ourselves. Three years after the research we managed to set up a project for a very personal, very club member-led type of centre where the facilitators were responsive to the stated wishes of the people attending the centre. So for once they had control. People were still saying, you have too highly qualified staff, an RMN G grade, a senior occupational therapist, and two care assistants for ten club members. Too many staff, too expensive. We held out and got what we wanted. We have ten relatively young people, aged from 40 to 65 years, very different individuals, with a whole variety of needs, not prepared to be herded into groups. So we do need four staff to give the members what they want. We can then spread our staff. Six months down the line we already have a long waiting list to join the club.

D: It is such a complex area of work. There shouldn't be any question but that you need very highly qualified staff . . . taking on virtually untrained care staff to work with people with such difficulties seems to be immoral, in my view. It is really good that you stuck out . . .

N: Something we have to learn is that, if you are in your seventies and eighties and have dementia, I am not saying that it less sad but you may have fulfilled a lot of what you want to do. We have had a lady of 39 at the centre and she has a lot of life yet to lead. She knew she was losing her memory. She has a husband, and a young child, and was worried about it being hereditary. And what affect was it going to have on him. She had her own parents to think about as well. A complex support system was needed. Our society is starting to offer counselling for dementia. One might ask, what is the point, but if it improves a person's quality of life, I don't care how long for, then that is the point.

D: I know you have been very supportive to the weekly art therapy group at the centre, which primarily attends to the quality of life, and to the loss, to the terrible sadness that people feel. In a way it is like the hospice movement has accepted that people dying of cancer can be helped by some form of therapy.

N: The normal sort of activity set up by day centres might help in the immediate now, but does it actually help for the future? My understanding is that people want to go to art therapy and I am told that the individuals who attend are more relaxed, calm, afterwards. They have a choice and they choose to go. It is about people's quality of life. I used to think back to the time when Aids became prevalent, and to the term 'living with Aids', and I now start to use the phrase 'living with dementia'. Certainly in working with younger people, they are very aware of their future, they don't need you to tell them. They want to get what they can out of life now.

D: I think one of the difficult things is the regimentation we were talking about, which seems still to be the case in a lot of places, and the lack of an opportunity to feel upset, grieved, to deal with sadness or loss.

N: In many day centres, staff feel they have failed if one of their residents sits and cries, and I say, no you have failed when you stop them crying. Why should they be jollied out of their feelings. You want someone to say, you are looking quite sad today, to acknowledge how you are and to talk with you. If art therapy is a way to get people to express how they are feeling, that is good.

D: The jolliness masks a terrible sadness and fear which is lurking underneath. It is difficult for the care workers because they can take in a lot of the projected feelings and they don't realise it, and then they burn out or get ill. There's a kind of hysterical merriment in some centres I have visited, contrasting with a paralysing inactivity on behalf of the residents . . .

N: It is important for care workers to have supervision, and we provide that in the Society. It is important to have access to support, because in this work you are a sponge and sponges, to be effective, have to be wrung out occasionally and unless you give support and supervision to staff you are putting an unfair burden on them. Also by giving support you are enabling a care worker to be very receptive to a client. If not you get bad practice. I am very keen that the health and social services continue our partnership, because you need a multitude of skilled staff, who can share their skills.

D: Not only in dementia care, this can be the way forward for any illness . . . especially in so-called mental illness . . . where a person can also lose their identity.

N: You can't divorce the physical from the social and spiritual . . .

D: I think the French, or at least it seems from their literature,[1] appear to be rather more in touch with the spiritual and psychological issues around dementia, the existential problems, whereas in the UK the emphasis seems to have been around 'managing' it, 'dealing' with it . . .

N: This shows more ability to be in touch with feelings around the condition.

D: I have had conversations with medical staff in the UK, where they have been adamant that there is no point having any psychological, or rather psychotherapeutic, input with people with dementia. That seems very strange . . .

N: It is, because dementia doesn't mean a blanket attack in one day! It is gradual, therefore it is affecting the inner person, their identity . . . and that has to be acknowledged.

D: The excuse given is that people with severe dementia don't have insight – but we can never really say how aware somebody is, how much insight they have – we don't know. They might not appear to be aware but then they may well be. I think Oliver Sacks's *Awakenings*[2] and Luria's *The Man with the Shattered Mind*[3] – who was apparently oblivious to everything around him, but actually wasn't – are remarkably valuable books for anyone trying to understand about dementia.

N: You can never say there is no psychological need. We need to be understood, be part of things, and if you ignore that you can exaggerate the distortions that dementia brings about.

D: And we don't know how much the culture of negativity and hopelessness has contibuted to people becoming very much worse than they need to be.

N: I am thinking about an elderly lady in a day centre, in an art therapy session, who was painting, very quietly, and she came out to see me afterwards. I said to her, did you find that useful, and she said, 'I can't say in words but that picture shows you how I feel.' Although I didn't understand the picture myself, I thought, if she feels she has communicated, felt it had been a step forward, then that was most important. On the other hand, there was a man who always painted very bleak pictures in an art class, but because this was in an activity session the staff didn't know what to do with him. I felt so sad, and that is probably why I wanted to bring in art therapy, because this man could have been helped in the torment going on in his mind. What was he thinking, what was happening . . .?

D: Sometimes the images from art therapy are very horrifying, very powerful, but in a way, if someone has been able to bring these feelings out, it could help them . . . For this man, in art therapy there is someone there to share his feelings . . .

N: Whereas in the art class, the staff really didn't know what to do about these terrifying paintings . . . they were asking, should we even allow him to come to the class, perhaps we are picking scabs off wounds . . . will it upset the others?

D: They obviously had a point because, although he needed to externalise what was going on, it would have been better if he had someone to receive it as well. That is one of the important things about art therapy, the receiving of feelings. That becomes part of the group culture – as opposed to stuffing down feelings and pretending to be jolly!

N: The work of the Towner Club art therapy group will hopefully show that there have been some positives. It might also point us to further developments.

D: Perhaps some individual sessions could be helpful, and maybe some provision for carers who are so loaded with guilt and dread. I wanted to include the term *Nameless Dread* in the title of this book, because I think dementia is a lot about living in a world which is full of dread. At least most of the time . . .

N: Isn't that a bit negative, or is that the theme you want to get across . . .?

D: Yes, I think the experience is of being in a world where you don't know what is going to happen, you can't put a name to it, it is living every day and night with a certain dread of what might happen. It is being in a state of complete terror. But you can't easily pin it down. It is paralysing, and it always struck me how the 'freezing' element of Parkinson's got worse at times of major confusion and apprehension. It is like looking at a wall when you can't differentiate what's there. I can look at that wall and see filing boxes up there, books, different colours, but if I looked at the wall and all I could see was a mass of things, undifferentiated, I wouldn't know where I was in the world. We have to accept this is happening when someone has dementia, but we can help it . . . It is awful . . . but we can do something. After all, having an illness such as terminal cancer is awful, but it doesn't mean we can't do anything positive and indeed we don't know how much positive we can do yet!

N: Until we know we can do something positive about dementia then people are not going to want to have a test, they are not going to want a diagnosis, so they will leave it too late till there is not much that can be done . . . it is difficult.

D: Do you think the title 'dementia', the name of the condition, is a problem in itself? I mean, the terms for mental illness and mental handicap have changed a lot . . . I get worried about these labels and how they determine what happens. I am absolutely sure that, except in exceptional circumstances, the label 'dementia' condemns people to a half-existence . . .

N: Our society has dropped the 'disease' from 'Alzheimer's disease'. At one time, when my grandmother had Alzheimer's, the GPs were hardly aware of it. Nowadays, anyone with signs of dementia has 'Alzheimer's' . . . it seems to be something more understood and even palatable to mention than 'dementia'. We could drop 'dementia', but can we think of another name which is not Alzheimer's? The Society thought about changing but felt that people now knew more about Alzheimer's. It may not be so connected with the notion of 'senile dementia' . . .

D: Yes, also with public figures like Iris Murdoch having Alzheimer's, and Ronald Reagan, there may be more awareness. But there are issues about the other dementias, and indeed other progressive illnesses. The Pope has Parkinson's (I would say he clearly has had it for a long time but it has only just been acknowledged), and Mohammed Ali definitely has. The moment when he got the Sportsman of the Century Award was so emotional. I know a lot of people were in tears, including myself. I wonder where people with other dementias, Parkinson's-related, Lewy Body and multi-infarct, for instance, would think to get support?

N: They probably wouldn't think to come to us, unless somebody has actually said, your husband has Parkinson's and as well has (dementia). They would probably assume they should go to the Parkinson's Society.

D: They probably would, and might think that they just had to get on with it, and it was what Parkinson's was about. To be fair I would imagine the PDS would give help if they knew someone had related dementia, or would refer them to the Alzheimer's Society. I hope so. So there is quite a bit of public education to do on the whole issue of what to do when someone starts showing signs of dementia . . .

N: It's like Aids-related dementia, not many people with Aids would turn to the Alzheimer's Society, yet 10 per cent of people with Aids can get dementia on UK figures. They do not tend to come to us.

D: The total horror, and I *am* going to call it *Nameless Dread*, is to do with the horror of the concept, the horror of the diagnosis and the descent into dread which has been reinforced by the lack of good person-centred care – there is no going away from the fact that if someone has dementia the prognosis is grim . . . images are still, usually, of the smelly, noisy, hopelessness of the geriatric ward . . . of which many still exist.

N: We need to have better awareness and information about some of the good things, the outings for example, that happen in our centres, so that the public at large know that people with dementia can still enjoy things like anyone else. We need to portray those images, rather than what is always shown in the media – diagnosis today, burn down the kitchen next week and into residential care.

D: I can remember when Dan had the diagnosis of Parkinson's he went immediately into a depression, so severe that he did not ever really come out of it. He felt it as a death sentence, in that he only had images of people shuffling and dribbling in geriatric wards. He saw that as the end. The consultant was most insensitive, pointing out to a group of medical students: Look, those are typical signs of Parkinson's . . . and on finding out I was a therapist, took delight in emphasising that 'it was not a psychosomatic illness'. When I expressed surprise that he had said that (as I had not mentioned it) he repeated himself. I said that surely psychological factors played a part in the course of the illness, which he rather dismissed. We were sent out with instructions to look up the number of the Parkinson's Society in the phone book! And an instruction to make an appointment with the GP. Thank God that the PDS were so responsive so quickly, and so was Dan's GP, otherwise we would both have become severely depressed. At that point he had mild Parkinson's and I had no idea that he was likely to develop dementia. Just as well.

N: The point at which diagnosis is given is so important and it is often overlooked, how devastating it can be.

D: You know very well what a fight it all was! But do you have any further thoughts now, any points you want to make?

N: We must start having a generally better quality of care, especially in residential homes, a better knowledge of dementia and time to put theoretical knowledge into practice. The care profession needs to be valued. Nobody would say that it is easy, working with people with dementia, so the staff need support and to feel part of a team. And a major change of attitude.

D: Maybe that will come with the new NHS document, *Making a Difference* – who knows? But until there is decent training, there is support, homes are not run for profit alone, and staff are not expected to 'baby sit' people with severe difficulties, twenty people with two members of staff, overworked, impossible . . .

N: Yes, and individual attention, because if I have dementia and I want to get up at 4 a.m. I should be able to. But if one member of staff is looking after thirty other people then there is no way I can. My frustration is, I go out to do training, then I find there aren't the resources for staff to put it into practice.

D: Well-trained staff and smaller numbers, and greater possibility for support for people to stay at home, with help. This comes at a cost, but we can afford it! Our society is rich and can afford it.[4]

N: We have to provide for it . . . in the same way as for physical care. It is no good having a new plastic hip joint if I am stuck in some awful place with no life. It's a question of priorities.

Notes

1 A particularly useful book for French speakers, which looks at dementia from a psychoanalytic–object relations perspective, is C. Montani (1994) *La Maladie d'Alzheimer: Quand la Psyche s'egare*, Paris: L'Harmatton.

2 See O. Sacks (1973) *Awakenings*, New York: HarperCollins, or the 1991 edition (London: Pan Books).

3 See A.R. Luria ([1968] 1987) *The Mind of a Mnemonist*; also *The Man with a Shattered Mind* ([1972] 1987), both Cambridge, Mass: Harvard University Press.

4 Shortly before submitting this book for publication, the government announced that Aricept and similar drugs could now be freely prescribed at a cost of approximately £45 million per annum; the following day Parliament resolved to allow research using tissue from embryos, with the aim of finding a cure for progressive illnesses such as Parkinson's and Alzheimer's.

Chapter 9

A narrowed sense of space

An art therapy group with young Alzheimer's sufferers

Barry Falk

Introduction

The term 'young Alzheimer's sufferers' refers to people below the age of 65. For this group of people, many of whom are still active and living at home, the onset of Alzheimer's raises a whole set of issues which need addressing.

'Until recently, there were virtually no services for this forgotten group.'[1]

The definition of dementia is 'a madness marked by failure or loss of mental powers, feeble-mindedness';[2] in fact another word for schizophrenia is 'dementia praecox'. Dementia is also a malady often associated with the elderly: 'senile dementia'. Formerly people over 65 with the associated symptoms were diagnosed as suffering from senile dementia and those below that age said to be suffering from pre-senile dementia. Senility has always referred to the dementia of old age. For young Alzheimer's sufferers, then, this label may be an embarrassing one to wear, a tag commonly associated with being old and being insane, none of which was an accurate description of the client group I was working with.

'Dementia is not a disease in itself but a group of symptoms that may accompany certain diseases. Alzheimer's disease is one of the most common causes of dementia.'[3]

The definition of both Alzheimer's and its ensuing dementia is often blurred, the latter often defining the former; there has in fact been an 'Alzheimerization'[4] of dementia. The danger is that the label defines the individual; as one group member put it: 'If we had red spots people would see that we were ill, but with this [Alzheimer's] people don't understand.' I feel it is important, therefore, to define clearly the specific issues which faced the client group that I was working with. The prevailing issues which came up were: of being confined, literally housebound; grief around the impending sense of loss;

frustration with being overly dependent upon help, and anxiety provoked by the disorientating effect of the disease.

The art therapy sessions were part of a wider project looking into the benefits of setting up a new and innovative service specifically for this client group. The aim of the 'club' was to provide a flexible service, meeting two days a week, and to therefore re-evaluate how the care services can best meet the needs of this largely 'forgotten' client group.

The staff team comprised a team leader, an occupational therapist, two support workers, myself (the art therapist), and a regular volunteer. The programme of activities on offer was flexible, drawing upon the requests and needs of those attending. The range of activities included dance and movement groups, walks, shopping trips, indoor activities and outdoor trips in a minibus. The people attending were referred to as 'club members', therefore seeking to reinforce the philosophy that they determine the culture of the centre.

The art therapy was included at the outset of the club, aiming to provide an additional therapeutic space. In order to create a safe space the art therapy group needed to establish a consistent meeting time and period of duration. At the time of writing the group had been running for forty sessions, thus establishing a continuity of presence within the club. During this time the set-up of the art therapy space had to adapt in order to establish clear boundaries and to define itself within the open-plan setting.

The aim of this study is to explore the benefits of this type of therapeutic activity with this particular client group within this type of day-care setting.

Setting up a safe space

The first few sessions were characterised by a general sense of disarray: staff interruptions, cigarette breaks and wandering attention. The level of anxiety felt particularly high within the art therapy group. The art therapy space was, at this time, an extension of the club meeting space; before the art therapy session the members and staff would all meet up to discuss the programme of events for the day and to allow a group feedback time. Once the meeting was over this space was then used for the art therapy. Members were given the choice as to whether they wanted to remain and participate, but the effect, I felt, of this shared-space arrangement was to create the sense of a captive audience. The anxiety of the new setting, I feel, made decision-making difficult and, subsequently, limited choice – the choice of whether to attend the art therapy or not. This was seen in the group by an initial resistance to using the art materials, a reluctance to move from the seated circle to explore the art table.

It was decided that the art therapy space and the club meeting space would be two different areas of the room, to differentiate them and create clearer boundaries. Outside interruptions, it was also agreed, would be minimised.

As the art therapy progressed, it was interesting to see what impact it had, if any, upon the members. A number of benefits did appear to accompany the art therapy process: a more focused attention span, within the group dialogue as well as during the art activity; a way of working through some of the stuckness, verbally and non-verbally; and the creation of a space, which, though confined, felt active and interactive.

By session five the group felt a lot more cohesive. Certain club members had decided they wouldn't attend the art therapy, and others were keen to attend. No longer were there mid-session cigarette breaks, and the group members seemed able to stay within the boundaries of the space for the duration of the session. This created a more focused and intimate group, which was beginning to establish what issues could be brought to the sessions and to explore the space via the art materials.

The Alzheimer's monster

The art activity threw up a great deal of themes and images. For Irene there was a preoccupation with monsters and large animals. In session one she was dying to tell us what Mandy's picture meant to her: 'It's a large dinosaur that swims underwater, lethal!' In session ten she told us that she could see 'a big animal with the word "Alzheimer's" written below it'. When asked to describe the big animal she got up and drew it with her hands. In session thirty Irene explained to Mia that when she draws 'this thing, I call it the Alzheimer's monster, always comes up, with his teeth'.

These images appeared to me to be vivid descriptions of her fears surrounding the Alzheimer's. Ofra Kamar, describing similar observations of a man suffering from Alzheimer's that he was working with, writes: 'Absorbed, Steve drew and drew, summoning up from his inner depths creatures that I later realised were metaphors for his fears and anxieties'.[5]

For Irene the art therapy tapped into a highly vivid imagination. Irene was taking Aricept medication; before this she would have periods of hallucinating. The art activity seemed to be tapping into this 'hallucinatory' imagination. Irene's first image was an intricate assemblage of symbols. As she explained: a snowman with a smiling face was 'the house'; two arrows connected to swirly marks, which resembled the shape of a brain, and which were 'all the confusion and darkness'; another arrow pointed to the words 'Hope, Peace and the World', which was about 'wishing peace upon the world'. She had also written the word 'SHALOM' below the snowman, and a small blue door above with the word 'ouch!' 'The doors are difficult to get through', she explained. In Irene's case the thoughts and images appeared to come through uninhibited.

For Irene, the artwork was self-revealing and allowed her space to make sense of her images/visions. For Tom, though, the art activity unlocked a box full of dread and fear. 'I always make horrible art', he told us. In session two

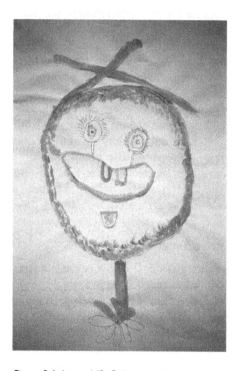

Figure 9.1 Irene. NB Colour versions of the figures in this chapter can be viewed at www.brunner-routledge.co.uk/WallerArtsTherapies

Tom drew five figures on hangman's nooses; there were five in his family. The expression of these horrible thoughts provoked a sad response in him, which was difficult to bear in the group. The sadness brought a caring response from Irene, but the rest of the group responded with awkward silence. The following week Tom left his artwork up at the table, preferring to keep his 'horrible thoughts' to himself. Tom refused to attend any more sessions, the feelings evoked in him seeming too unbearable to bring safely to the art therapy group.

By bringing together a group of young Alzheimer's sufferers, the club also served as a stark reminder of the debilitating effect of the disease. Within the art therapy session this contrast was heightened. Lucy joined the group in session five. She was the youngest club member and had been diagnosed with a much more rapidly deteriorating form of dementia. In session five Lucy painted a blue sweeping shape, which she told us was 'a warrior ship'; she told us she intended to 'fight it'. Lucy expressed a lot of anger within the sessions, anger with herself for being 'a failure'. The anger she felt was transferred into this spirited image of a 'warrior ship'. In session seven she inadvertently poured green paint over Mandy's picture; she told us she'd wanted to make a

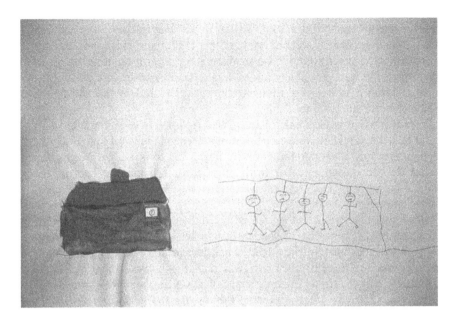

Figure 9.2 Tom

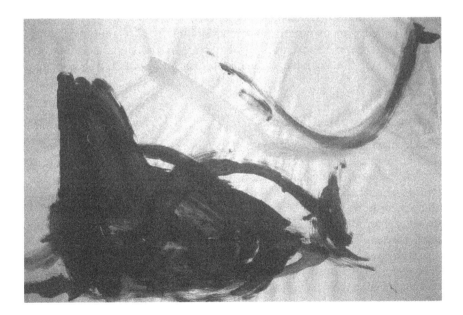

Figure 9.3 Lucy

mess, though she didn't normally feel like this. In session ten she was exasperated, repeatedly saying 'I don't know what to do.' Her image of two abstract shapes, one quite heavily worked on, the other lighter and more spontaneous in appearance, seemed to me to be expressing her separation anxiety. In session twelve she was very shaky and it was difficult to calm her down. The close attention of the group, though, contained her and by the end of the session she said she felt a lot calmer.

There was a two-week break for Lucy, who returned in session fifteen. This would be her last session, as a care home had been arranged for her to stay at, the option of her staying at home was no longer felt to be viable. During this session another group member, with more chronic dementia, became the focus of concern for Lucy, appearing to mirror her own fears and anxieties about the effects of the disease.

Lucy's rapid deterioration presented the difficult issue, for the others, of seeing the debilitating effect of the dementia reflected in a much starker manner. Over the sessions that she attended her deterioration was very apparent. The real fear for the club members was their inevitable decline in health: 'Eventually people with Alzheimer's completely lose the ability to care for themselves ... In the latest stages of the disease the brain can no longer regulate body functions and victims die of malnutrition, dehydration, infection, heart failure or other complications'.[6] In session twenty-eight, Irene told me about a meeting she'd had the day before with a counsellor, at a hospital for elderly mentally ill patients. The theme of the meeting had been about planning for the future; the implication, Irene told me, was of going into care. The picture she drew was shocking: a figure with no arms or legs, just a flower stem for a body, an inane grin and mad-looking eyes; it appeared quite insane. Irene appeared shaken up by her picture and of the implication of going 'mad'; the unbearable thought of losing control and becoming institutionalised.

A narrowed sense of space

A noticeable feature of some of the club members was often a disconnected, flat look, suggesting a depressed, non-interactive state. Depression, which is a common symptom of dementia, exacerbated by the difficulty to articulate verbally, could be easily misinterpreted as reflecting an inability to make cognitive decisions or to understand (bearing in mind the etymological link between the words 'dementia' and 'madness').[7] Yet this state of apparent stuckness could be changed, as was demonstrated in the art therapy and also in the club in general – the real person allowed to express themselves.

The depressed self also suggested, to me, a defensive stance which, I felt, reflected a need to detach emotionally from an environment which no longer made sense and was thus anxiety provoking, and in which they could no longer participate. For the club members the external world had become a confusing place where the road signs no longer correlated; space had, literally, become confined. The analogy could be made that a narrowed sense of space was a reflection of the self in a state of disarray.

In session two Tom drew a picture of a house with a person looking out of the window. He explained that he was this person stuck inside the house: 'If I go outside I get lost.' His house had no door and only one window. There was a strong feeling of confinement and of being alone. Tom's image of the house and being stuck inside resonated with the other group members. The house as a symbol of self was an image that often came up. In session thirty-one Irene told us about the builders coming into her home and of the family having to move to temporary accommodation for a few weeks. Irene described the house now as being 'all stripped bare, you can hear your voice echo'. Her drawing was even more revealing: 'This is my house and this black mark is all the dust; it's really nasty stuff. And these are my weak legs; I'm trying to carry it all.' She admitted that, 'Really, I'm going to pieces', which reflected what was literally happening to her home. The repercussions, for Irene, of having builders come in to do major restructuring work, was the loss of a secure base, exacerbated by the already disorientating effect of the Alzheimer's disease.

For many of the members, still relatively young and physically active, the response to their feeling of confinement was to test the safe boundaries, to go for a wander. Ernest described one occasion when he went 'walkabout'. It was evening and he hadn't told his family he was going out: 'Well, they were all in there talking and I was washing up and I thought they could help me [to wash up]. So I went for a walk.' The nocturnal scene he described, sounded, as Irene said, 'spooky'; a place of darkness, disorientation and panic. It highlighted the dilemma for the members, struggling with their wish to retain independence yet not feeling safe enough to maintain this: their reliance upon a safe place yet the frustration with being confined.

The limited sense of space was reflected by the actual art therapy space: an area demarcated by low screens, within the larger open-plan club area. This presented the problem of outside interruptions, creating the sense of a loosely boundaried space. People had to walk by the group to get their coats or to go to the toilet. The table, therefore, became the holding space, with the art materials arranged in the centre. There was often a reluctance to explore the art materials, which reflected the muddling effect of the dementia but could also be seen as a reflection of the lack of clear boundaries: the open-plan setting raising the question of how safe was it to explore without straying away. Creating a safe holding-space therefore required my consistent presence and attention.

Within the countertransference this evoked a feeling of claustrophobia and anxiety, of frustration and the inability to concentrate. The fear was that I could not contain the group; that is, that I could not contain the high level of anxiety, the wandering attention and muddled thoughts. Added to this was the countertransference of working with a client group with a degenerative illness, the feelings of futility and lethargy. This was then projected out into the club: frustration with staff for allowing disruptions; the idea that I was overlooked/not being taken seriously/not respected; and the apprehension that the art therapy was resented by other staff members. Despite attending team meetings and expressing my concerns, these feelings were persistent and, I felt, mirrored what many of the members were experiencing.

A move towards an isolated place

'A narrowed sense of space' could also be interpreted as a euphemism for death. In session ten Irene told us about a funeral she'd been to the previous week. Describing the lowering of the coffin, she told us that 'the hole was so deep'.

Thomas recollected seeing his uncle die in a hospice: 'It was a horrible experience, he was all shaking. I wouldn't want to repeat that.' Thomas's painting, he explained, was of a view from his sister-in-law's flat, of a sunset over the sea. I noted that the houses, painted in silhouette, resembled tombstones; the whole image resonated with the theme of death, the theme of the session.

Thomas was one of the youngest club members. He was a regular group member for the first eighteen sessions. He normally presented as relaxed and

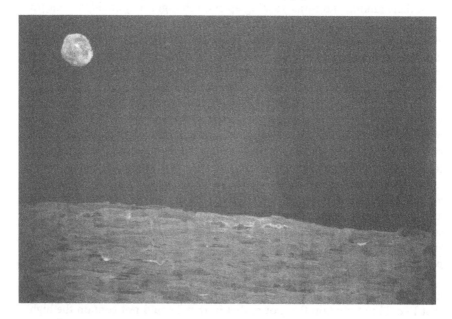

Figure 9.4 Thomas

jovial. He told us that he'd lost a lot of his social group now that he had Alzheimer's. He'd also lost a lot of the abilities, such as driving, cooking, getting out, which allowed him his independence. During the time he attended the group, though, he built up a rich body of work. Of a desert scene he said, 'It's a place where I can go to be alone.' Thomas was expressing the need to take himself to a quieter place, literally painting himself into a space free from disturbance. The need for solitude related, I felt, to his need to re-establish a sense of self; the art activity seemed to offer him a place of refuge, providing an internal space in which he could find himself again. It connected, I felt, to Ernest's urge to go 'walkabout': the need to reassert a sense of independence.

The images which Thomas made were often stark in appearance: desolate, isolated places. In my mind they suggested a move towards separation; an acknowledgement of endings, of death. I also felt that they were exploring the idea of defacement, of a sense of self made desolate by the dementia. In session twelve Thomas made a small clay head. Irene pointed out that it looked like a skull. Thomas said he'd got the idea for his sculpture from watching a television programme about temples in Cambodia, 'where the faces had been defaced'. Thomas referred to his sculpture as his 'boogalloo'. The group discussed Thomas's boogalloo; Irene said it was about fear and Lucy said *they* didn't understand. The underlying theme seemed to me to be about the loss of identity caused by the dementia. The boogalloo had been defaced and lost in the jungle.

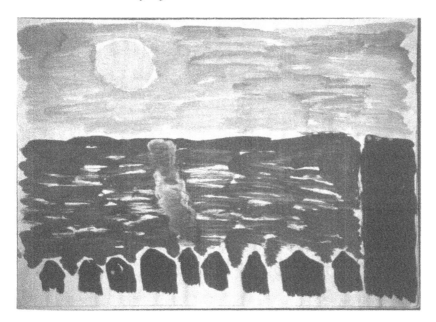

Figure 9.5 Thomas

An interior holding-space

Each group member had their idiosyncratic way of working, from Irene's complex images to Lucy's looser abstract pieces. Over the course of the sessions a rich dialogue was created around the images, which often resonated around the group and fed into the dialogue. The images provided a focus which held the group's attention, communicating ideas and feelings which were not being verbally expressed and also acting as an important holding-space.

Maddy joined the group in session three. She presented as always active and outspoken, often impulsive, with a short attention span; quick to start talking with people but her conversation in the nature of a soliloquy. Verbally her speech was flighty and seemingly muddled; she would often mix up her tenses, so that events that were in the future were spoken about in past tense, and vice versa. The content of her speech was interesting: natural disasters and things in states of disarray were often spoken about, and often insightful, though blunt, observations of other group members peppered her monologue. She appeared to pay little attention to the verbal responses of others, seemingly wrapped up in her own preoccupations. Interestingly, though, the non-verbal art activity focused her attention. Once at the art table, with paper and art materials at hand, she would paint for up to an hour or more, completely absorbed in the activity. Her images remained consistent – she appeared to have a number of favourite themes: a boat and kite scene, a

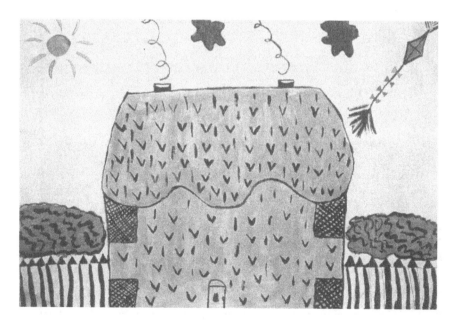

Figure 9.6 Maddy

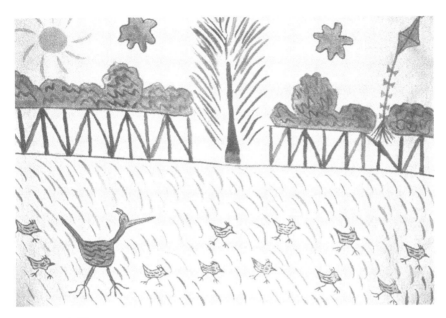

Figure 9.7 Maddy

cottage scene, and a pond and birds scene. She also seemed to come to the group with an image in mind, which she would first sketch out and then methodically colour in with watercolour paints. Her images were bright and active; as one group member commented in response to one picture: 'It's amazing. It makes me feel happy.' Once the activity was finished, though, she would talk over others and soon wander off from the group.

The art activity offered the opportunity for Maddy to enter an active, symbolic space. The images were repetitive and the dialogue around the themes limited. Yet they defined an area of play and interest which Maddy appeared to derive a great deal of satisfaction from; places where she felt alive and active.

As well as providing a place of refuge, the art activity allowed a space in which to feel alive. Dorothy explained to the group that her first picture was 'going for a walk on the Downs'. Watching her paint it did feel like she had gone for a tentative walk across the paper, exploring the space. As the sessions continued she begun to explore the area of the paper more. She seemed to be mapping the space, finding out how far she could go in one direction how far in the other. The types of art material she chose also affected how quickly, how far, she could move. Dorothy expressed her frustration with one picture which she had been working on over four sessions. She had been using light pencils on a dark background; the image only covered a fifth of the paper and was difficult to distinguish. She admitted to me that she felt stuck and decided

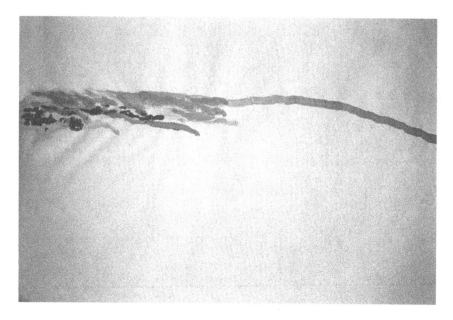

Figure 9.8 Dorothy

that the following week she would start a new picture. In fact it wasn't until three sessions later (due to absence from the group) that she began a new picture, but she remembered clearly her desire to start something new. Using felt-tip pens she worked quite quickly, covering the whole sheet of paper with different colours. This change of art materials felt like a breakthrough for her. She described her picture as: 'a kitten pushing over balls of wool'. The idea of woolliness seemed pertinent to suffering from Alzheimer's, but more importantly, I felt, the image was playful and exploratory.

For Dorothy the artwork also acted as a holding-memory; she would often return to pieces started the previous week. Within the arena of the paper, the art activity, Dorothy was able to explore and challenge her boundaries; despite her expressed wish to 'make a mess' she normally worked slowly and carefully. The artwork, in fact, highlighted her limitations, yet also offered the potential to create something new. Although Dorothy accepted assistance there was an insistence on her part that she worked at her own pace, 'muddling' her way through.

The question comes to mind of what happens to the sense of the self when the effects of the Alzheimer's takes hold. Winnicott explained that 'in healthy development, the developing child becomes autonomous, and becomes able to take responsibility for himself or herself independently of highly adapted ego support'.[8] It seems to me that what Winnicott is talking about is the development of an *interior holding-space*, a *mirroring*, for the child, of the

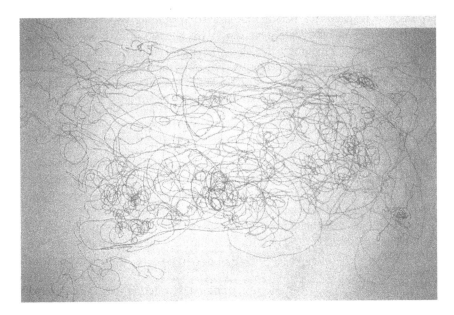

Figure 9.9 Dorothy

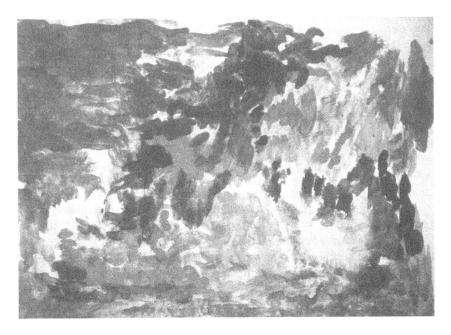

Figure 9.10 Dorothy

maternal holding. He goes on to say that 'In so far as the individual boy or girl has now reached to a personal organisation of inner psychic reality, this inner reality is constantly being matched with samples of external or shared reality.' For the club members this ability to organise an inner psychic reality was being destroyed by the degenerative effects of the disease. The art therapy was able to assist the group members to re-establish a sense of a holding-space within which they could re-establish a sense of self.

Conclusion

The effects of Alzheimer's is a loss of spatial orientation and a reduced ability for abstract thought. Curiously, though, the imagination often appears to become heightened, not hampered, by the dementia. This increased imagination, akin to free association, can be linked to the symptoms of the disease: 'Many people with Alzheimer's disease experience psychotic symptoms with the advancing severity . . . The most common of these symptoms include paranoid delusions . . . misidentification syndromes . . . and hallucinatory experiences'.[9]

The question that arose in my mind was whether the art therapy process was beneficial or whether it exacerbated the sense of helplessness and encouraged the hallucinations, thus encouraging the 'madness'?

For different group members the effects of the dementia varied; as many variables, in fact, as personalities. Subsequently the artwork and art activity varied, ranging from complex, highly symbolic images to loosely abstract pieces. For all of them, though, it offered a safe place within which to bring and explore complex and difficult thoughts and feelings. The therapeutic value of the art lay, therefore, in its role of providing a means of communication when verbal articulation was often very difficult, or impossible.

The symbolic images also acted as a strong holding-memory. A capacity to hold them in mind, from week to week, was often demonstrated, when many of the other details of the day had been forgotten. Perhaps what was being demonstrated was a necessary move from an exterior space, that was perceived as muddled and full of dread, to an interior space, over which they had some sense of control. The artwork provided a holding-memory, a tangible object to look back upon, but also a symbolic memory which appeared to be more easily retained.

Despite the lack of clear boundaries around the art therapy area, the 'ritual deconstruction' of the art therapy space at the end of the session exposing the illusion, the art therapy was maintained, and as the sessions went on the group members' ability to stay for the duration increased, which suggested that an interior holding-space was being created within the sessions and subsequently within their minds.

References

1 'A fresh approach to dementia' – 'trust talk': A newsletter for staff in the community mental health and rehabilitation services, South Downs Health, issue 90, May 2000.

2 Garmonsay, G.N. (1979) *The Penguin English Dictionary* (3rd edition), Harmondsworth: Penguin Books.

3 'A fresh approach to dementia' – 'trust talk': A newsletter for staff in the community mental health and rehabilitation services, South Downs Health, issue 90, May 2000.

4 Kitwood, T. (1997) *Dementia Reconsidered – The Person Comes First*, Buckingham/Philadelphia: Open University Press, p. 22.

5 Kamar, O. (1997) 'Light and death: art therapy with a patient with Alzheimer's disease', *American Journal of Art Therapy* 35: 120–121.

6 Cutler, N.R. and Sramek, J.J. (1996) *Understanding Alzheimer's Disease*, University Press of Mississippi, pp. xi.

7 Cutler and Sramek, op. cit., pp. xi.

8 Winnicott, D.W. (1971) *Playing and Reality*, London and New York: Routledge, pp. 130–131.

9 Heston, L.L. and White, J.A. (1991) *The Vanishing Mind: A Practical Guide to Alzheimer's Disease and Other Dementias*, New York: W.H. Freeman & Co., p. xiv.

Chapter 10

Evaluating the use of art therapy for older people with dementia

A control group study

Diane Waller

This chapter describes a multidisciplinary pilot project using two art therapy groups and two controls of ten weeks each (and the beginnings of a new follow-up project), to evaluate the effects of art therapy on a group of patients with dementia. It took place within Brighton Health Care Trust and was generously funded by the Alzheimer's Disease Society. It is the first completed art therapy study to use control groups.

This study compared an unselected group of volunteer patients with dementia who participated in art therapy sessions with a similar unselected group taking part in small group work facilitated by a senior care worker or occupational therapist. Both groups were assessed over ten sessions on measures of cognitive, behavioural and functional abilities.

The study found that people with dementia do respond to art therapy, as evidenced by decreased scores on an objective measure of depression. In addition to the depression scales, individuals clearly responded, as shown by the observer-rated mood changes reported within sessions. The outcome was encouraging enough to warrant further research and on 1 October 2000 the same team began a new, longer-term project funded for two years by PPP (Private Patient Plan) Health Care Trust. The current project builds on the knowledge gained from the pilot and it is extended to four art therapy groups and four controls, each lasting for nine months.

Background to the project

As other writers in this book have acknowledged, the fact that there are so many older people needing long-term care throughout health services world-wide cannot fail to be of deep concern to all of us. To provide an environment that promotes optimum health for the many physical and cognitive impairments experienced by this age group is a challenge to any health care provider's wisdom and creativity. It is of particular concern that many elderly people will suffer from forms of dementia, leading to a severe decline in mental abilities – most markedly in language, judgement, reasoning and memory.

For several years many art therapists have observed that people with dementia benefit from participation in art therapy sessions, but were not able to demonstrate this through systematic research. We had to rely on case study material and anecdotal evidence – and on the evidence which our patients could give us themselves, which, although meaningful to us, did not provide a base from which we could develop services and hence try to improve the care and quality of their lives. The few existing studies on art therapy with dementia patients have tended to appraise the effects on individuals; they have not been able to separate the effects of misdiagnosis, secondary illnesses, depression, poor drug management or general improvements in health care as major contributing variables (see Sheppard *et al.*, 1998). Studies which have evaluated art therapy and included older people with dementia argue that it provides a medium for emotional expression, an opportunity for reduction of social isolation and an environment where autonomy and choice may still be available (Spaniol, 1997; Shore, 1997; Beaujohn-Couch, 1997; Doric-Henry, 1997). Art therapy has the potential to enable expression and communication which could affect the behaviour of the patient during the session and also after. It may be that if the improvements within the group are able to be carried outside the session, it would also help carers and staff to be with the person with dementia with less stress and frustration all round.

As we have said before, a culture of hopelessness and despair is commonplace, though it is often hidden under a compensatory 'positive' attitude of staff and carers which leaves little room for patients to express their deep sadness at the losses they were experiencing: of cognitive abilities, relationships, freedom to move and live without being dependent on others. We have seen patients become increasingly frustrated and angry at not being able to express themselves adequately, and once lively and articulate people withdraw into passive, resentful muteness. Many activities offered in day centres and hospitals appear to be low-level and demeaning, and highlight a person's diminishing capabilities. Life loses its meaning.

Following the launch of a report on the particular problems of patients and carers with early onset dementia (as referred to by Neil McArthur in his interview, p. 100), it became evident that action could be taken to alleviate some of our disatisfaction with this state of affairs. As a result, Dr Jennifer Rusted, an experimental psychologist who had been a principal investigator on the above project, and myself, an art therapist and group analyst, joined with Linda Sheppard, a psychologist and researcher, Kim Shamash, a consultant psychiatrist with responsibility for elderly mentally ill, and Finlay McInally, an art therapist working in the local NHS Trust in Brighton, and together we devised a new project.

The aim was to evaluate objectively the effects of art therapy on a small number of people with dementia (these included people with Alzheimer's, advanced Parkinson's and multi-infarct dementia), using both quantitative and qualitative measures drawn from psychiatry, psychology and art therapy. The patients in the art therapy groups were compared with others who participated in control groups with a qualified health care professional. The patients were selected for the research project itself on the basis of their diagnosis and agreement to participate. Their agreement was felt to be extremely important, and, despite their having limited speech and possibly limited understanding, we wanted to put across exactly what would be involved and that attendance was absolutely voluntary. Their average age was 75. There were two art therapy groups, lasting ten weeks each, conducted at similar centres for the elderly, and two matched control groups. Our intention was to capture any changes in behaviour, cognition or mood and to analyse the resulting data by group and by individuals in the group. Ten weeks is a short period for any real benefit to accrue, but we felt this would enable us to assess whether or not patients might benefit from future involvement with art therapy as well as enabling us to observe the outcome systematically.

The cognitive tests used were the Mini-Mental State Exam, a brief measure of cognitive ability and two sub-tests (measuring sustained attention and visual selective attention) from the Test of Everyday Attention. Behavioural changes at a functional level were determined by staff observations using the Clifton Assessment Procedures for the Elderly (CAPE). Levels of depression were evaluated using the Cornell Scale for Depression in Dementia (CSDD). Physiological changes that affect activities of daily living were assessed using staff observations via the Barthel Activities of Daily Living. An adapted version of the Bond–Lader Mood Scale focusing on alertness, contentedness and sociability was used by the senior art therapist to assess the change in mood of the clients from the beginning to the end of the session. A further measure was implemented using the Carers Impression Based Interview (CIBI). This was obtained from the next of kin of each client or a separate staff member involved closely with that client.

Tests were carried out by Linda Sheppard, the research psychologist, at regular intervals throughout the ten weeks and for one month after. The art therapist, Finlay McInally, kept detailed case notes, together with photographs of the art work, which were monitored by myself, and this assessment was also submitted for inclusion in the report written up by Linda Sheppard and ourselves at the end of the project.

The art therapist was asked to identify people who had responded to art therapy two months after the staff observations were completed, and the therapist's assessment was submitted for inclusion in the final report. The data from these individuals was compared to the data collected from the control group and showed a marked difference in levels of depression between those that responded to art therapy and the control group. The difference was shown in a decreased level of depression for the responders from observations taken at commencement, mid-point and one month after follow-up (see Sheppard *et al.*, 1998).

Context

The groups took place in two day centres in Brighton, a city on the south coast of England, and they were matched as far as possible in terms of the services they provided, facilities and willingness to participate. We had to rely on the goodwill of staff in these institutions, none of whom had much prior knowledge of art therapy, although both the centres had painting or craft sessions run by care staff. The co-operation of the staff was essential in contributing to the assessment of patients during the period of the project and in supporting the groups.

The methodological problems of a project attempting to measure group effectiveness are considerable, and have been acknowledged particularly by Yalom (1983) in *In-Patient Group Psychotherapy*. Ensuring that the conditions of the researched group and the control are strictly maintained by the therapists, the co-worker and fellow workers preoccupied the research team throughout. We have to say that the only consistent factor was the art therapist, and it appeared to us that the variations in the context played an important part in determining the stability and effectiveness of the groups, and their benefit for patients.

We took this into account in preparing our longer-term project. For example, in institution (a) where time boundaries were carefully observed, the group 'gelled' over the ten-week period. The group appeared to be valued by other staff; the assistant therapist was present throughout and maintained an appropriate stance within the sessions. In the other institution (b) there was evidence of ambivalence towards art therapy. For example, the assistant therapist absented himself for two weeks without notice, with the permission of the line manager, who failed to inform the art therapist. This affected how the patients responded to the art therapy group; that is, they appeared reluctant to attend and anxious.

Communication within this group was affected by the ambivalence, which in turn was reflected in the way the patients used the materials and related to the therapist and each other.

In the supported group (a) the 'group cohesion' enabled patients to trust the process and resulted in a freer and richer use of materials. In one group there was evidence of carer ambivalence – for example, one patient went unexpectedly on respite for three weeks, another was taken shopping at the time of the group. We might speculate that carer ambivalence did not significantly affect the group process, whereas it did affect the individuals.

As to the environment, we had noted prior to commencing the project that the facilities in the two institutions were markedly different: in the first (a) there was a dedicated art and craft room, which easily accommodated up to six patients. It was well used, with plenty of materials available. There was no problem in acquiring extra materials and a locked cupboard for storage. In institution (b) the art room was very small and rarely used. A conservatory had to be converted each week prior to commencing the group. It had three different entrances, including one into the garden and was overlooked. It was on occasions very hot. There were few materials and the art therapist was obliged to purchase materials from the project budget. A locked cupboard was made available on the floor above.

In summary, the important contextual issues to emerge were about time and boundary maintenance in the groups, physical environment – such as a well-lit and ventilated room with plenty of materials – and staff attitude. Where these elements were positive, patients attended more regularly and showed greater improvement overall. Ambivalence among the staff team affected how the patients responded to the art therapy group; that is, patients were reluctant to attend and anxious. This reminded us that in any future project we would need to prepare staff much more thoroughly before starting the research and maintain closer contact throughout.

Summary of the groups

Note: names have been changed to maintain confidentiality.

In both groups the consistency of time and place, and the presence of the art therapist, enabled a group identity to form: some patients responded to this by attending, others by choosing to be absent.

For example: Thomas used clay to make an elephant and the following week Betty, on walking into the room, commented on the lumps of clay: 'It looks as if an elephant has been in here.' This suggests a sense of continuity. We noticed that patients were able to remember events and objects from week to week.

At the beginning the theme of being back at school was strong, in relation to the art materials. Art had not always been a positive experience and the sessions reminded the patients how they felt now – like children. The men viewed art as a not very worthwhile activity, more as something for girls or women, so, especially for the men, it was hard to allow themselves to play, rather than work. Work assumed great importance for the men. Terrance and Jack used the art materials to re-enact their previous identities, as a building manager and coalman respectively. When the patients were able to play in the sessions, they were able to let go of their identity: for example, Mathew was able to let himself be dependent rather than the 'family breadwinner', a note which had put him under great stress.

Gender roles were important, patients had a deep-rooted sense of what was masculine and what was feminine behaviour. The men were more dominant and fearful of giving up their roles. For example, Oliver needed to hold on to his identity through bringing in his daily newspaper and doing the crossword, as he had always done before. He became very involved in the group through using clay to make a car, to which he returned every week (Figure 10.1). This car seemed to symbolise his wish to retain some control over his life, and at

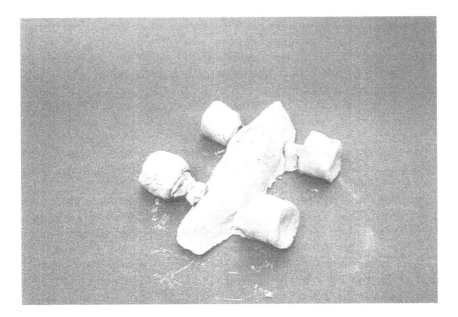

Figure 10.1

the same time he could mourn the fact that he could no longer drive, this being taken over by his wife. The dementia had robbed him of his retirement years and he urgently needed to escape from his predicament. He remembered his car from week to week and wished to continue with art therapy when the group's ten-week period came to an end.

The women in the group seemed more preoccupied with domesticity and caring roles, perhaps reflecting their age. Age was a very important issue. Several patients thought it was pointless being part of a group: they were 'too old'. We wondered if the 'pointlessness' was also picked up from the carers (is there any point in art therapy?), but we felt it was important that they could express this as it might have been an antidote to the culture of 'positive caring' where there was little room for expressions of negativity. The sense of 'filling the gaps while waiting to die' was strong. For example: Thomas didn't attend because he had 'too much to do'. By 'keeping busy' he could avoid despair. There was a strong sense of fear of dementia and dying, and powerful indications of loss.

How some of the patients used the group

Sylvia was cautious and feared having choices. She seemed imprisoned by a social role and by others' expectations of how women should behave. She was resistant to engaging with materials, and did not want to be persuaded into creating anything. She wasn't motivated, was depressed and bored and she said 'nothing particularly interested her'. It was important that she held on to her dignity. She eventually drew ticks on a sheet of paper, ticking off days, like waiting for a prison sentence to end. She was afraid of getting close to anyone. In the seventh session she drew a rainbow with a pot of gold at the end, where there was a life without depression, a magical place. She began to show interest, especially in Oliver's car. We felt that Sylvia was beginning to use the group and could have benefited from more time to get adjusted to being there.

Kate used the art materials as if she was cooking, and the table was a dining table. It felt as if she was trying to regain her role as housewife and mother. She often tasted and tried to eat the clay.

Deirdre needed to keep up appearances, to retain her identity as an active person with hobbies. During the group she became more playful and also expressed aggression and anger at her losses and being treated like a child. The clay pig (Figure 10.2) that she made was, she felt, ugly and dirty, like the clay and perhaps like herself, in her eyes. She used clay to explore her relationship with her recently deceased husband, and also made a dolphin (Figure 10.3), which could symbolise wanting to be rescued. The art therapy group helped her to express deep feelings of loss and despair.

Oliver needed to hold on to his identity through bringing in his *Times* newspaper and doing the crossword. He was engaged in the group especially

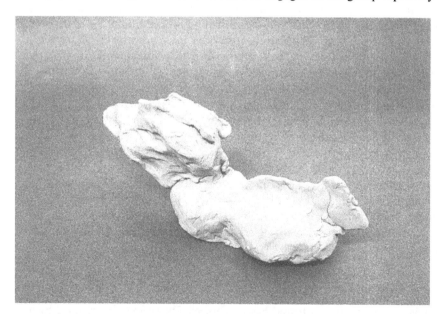

Figure 10.2

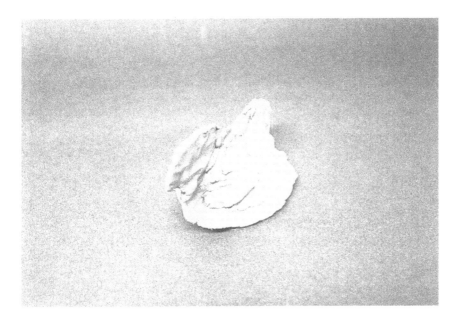

Figure 10.3

through making a car out of clay, to which he returned every week. His progress was interrupted by an unplanned three-week respite organised by his wife. The car seemed to symbolise his wish to retain some potency, and at the same time he mourned the loss of his driving ability (his wife had to drive for him). The Parkinson's had robbed him of his retirement years and left him needing to escape from his predicament. He remembered his car from week to week and at the end of the group wished to continue with art therapy.

Jack needed to hold on to his work identity, when he had been a coalman. He also experienced loss of sexual potency and was troubled by a catheter. He felt art was for children and women and that he was too old and there was no point. He squeezed his image into the corner of the paper as if he had no right to be anywhere else. He was threatened by Oliver, who was more able, and so retained some energy in competition with him.

Thomas felt he was not being told the truth, being patronised and manipulated. He seemed to experience the group as a negative place and felt that the art was for children. It was paradoxically interesting that he attended, and was able to express his anger and irritation while in the group.

Betty used the clay and was able to express some humour; for example by making 'elephant turds' (Figure 10.4). She became more animated whilst using clay. When one of the men criticised her drawing she was able to get angry with him, but quickly became powerless and deflated. She used the clay

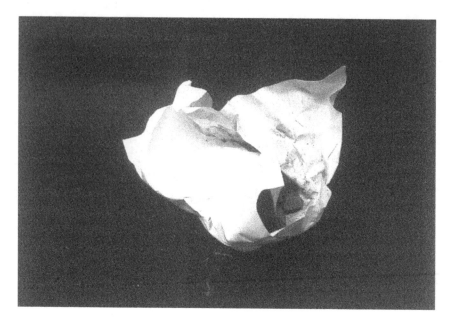

Figure 10.4

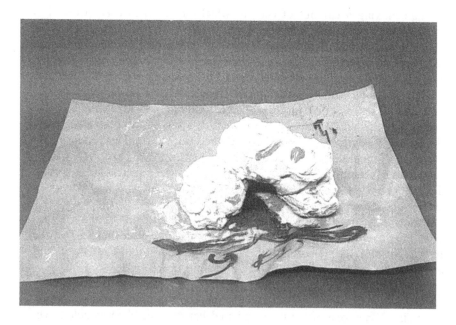

Figure 10.5

to make a cave 'where children play', which was womb-like (Figure 10.5). She seemed to experience the group as a safe place.

Terrance needed to hold things together. He had been in a high-up position in the building trade and felt responsible for everyone. He couldn't allow himself to feel dependent. He wanted to make order out of chaos. He was critical and controlling of one of the women and treated her like a child. He interacted energetically, but with some hostility – especially to women. He made a clay elephant (Figure 10.6).

Arthur was very interested in the art materials and in the quality of the paper. His interest in frames, which he drew on a large sheet of paper (Figure 10.7), suggested a need for containment. He feared messy materials. He needed rules and control and to be dominant in the group. The art materials reminded him of his losses (for example, his art college experience); he had not been involved with art since his dementia began. He found it difficult to let go emotionally or symbolically. To Arthur the frame was more important that what was in it. He seemed to fear the commitment and intimacy of being in the group. Nevertheless, with time, art therapy might allow him to let go and become less fearful.

These descriptions cannot really express the wealth of interactions in the groups and the powerful, often painful, but also humorous, moments over the ten weeks. Finlay McInally's account of part of a session within one of the groups gives an idea of what it was like (see the Case vignette, pp. 134–136).

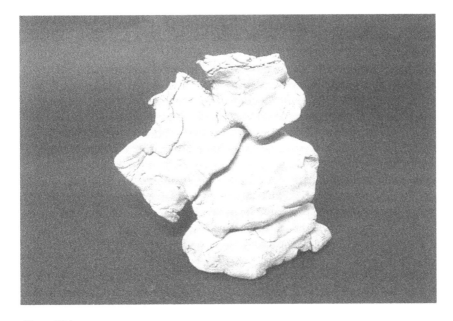

Figure 10.6

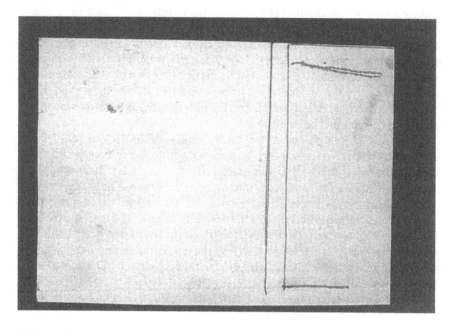

Figure 10.7

Results

Following the battery of cognitive tests and observational assessments which were carried out by independent raters, we were able to show that people with dementia do respond to art therapy, as evidenced by decreased levels of depression and improved mood of the individuals in the group. Given the brevity of the project, and the fact that the patients had been randomly assigned to art therapy, these findings seemed quite remarkable and encouraged us to design a further control study over a longer period of time. The ten-week groups enabled us to assess whether or not the patients could benefit from further involvement with a consistent and well-supported art therapy experience. The normal length of such a group would be about a year, and, given the patient group's particular needs, it would seem that having a slow-open group with this lifespan could be of benefit to most of the patients who attended. We emphasised that this would need to be thoroughly supported by the institution that hosted the group, and staff therein would need to be prepared beforehand.

Following the preparation and publication of the pilot report and its distribution by the Alzheimer's Society in Brighton, we had much interest and feedback on the project, though sadly the promised additional art therapy sessions for patients who had benefited from the groups did not materialise. It seemed very important to carry on, so Jenny Rusted and I reviewed the experience and the outcome, and prepared a proposal for the next phase of the project. This time we balanced the qualitative and quantitive aspects, as we realised we had given more weight to the latter in the pilot. In order to test our initial findings and to see if the benefits would be replicated, or if other benefits or indeed the opposite would be shown, we proposed four art therapy groups and four controls, running for nine months each in four different institutions. Each group would have five or six patients with a diagnosis of moderate to severe dementia; the art therapy groups would be run by two qualified art therapists (two groups each) and an assistant, and the control groups (activity groups) by occupational therapists and assistants. The patients would not be on Aricept or other similar drugs, nor would they be engaging in other research projects. We budgeted to pay the therapists and assistants at the usual NHS scales, and for a full-time research assistant as manager of the project; we also organised funding for supervision of the art therapists and technical assistance. We aimed to keep the same team, with Dr Kim Shamash as consultant, bringing in Barry Falk, an art therapist qualified in work with dementia patients, and one or two occupational therapists and assistants employed specifically for the project. Jenny Rusted and myself would remain principal investigators with responsibility for different aspects of the work. We were thus delighted when PPP Health Care Trust funded our project, and work commenced on 1 October 2000. At the time of writing we are well on schedule, with all groups having started. Because this time round we had the benefit of our experience from the pilot, and appropriate funding, we were able to be very selective in our choice of institutions, in preparation of staff, and in preparation of the therapists. We have also realised how challenging it is to work in a multidisciplinary team, where the researchers come from such different disciplines as experimental psychology and art therapy, and this is an added benefit of the project for ourselves: we are united in our wish to 'make a difference' in this area, so we have brought all our skills together and challenged ourselves at the same time. We have undertaken the extended project with some trepidation, worrying in case, perhaps, we record no benefits in our final outcome. We don't believe that will be so, but the whole point of this systematic research is to put our hypothesis to the test. Whatever the outcome, the wealth of material generated by the careful recording of the individuals' interactions, the group process and the art works themselves over such a long period will provide a unique database. The methodology is rigorous and unusual in its balance of qualitative and quantitative aspects, and could easily be applied in other situations and with other patient groups. The findings of Yalom and others concerning the need for services to be well-supported within institutions in order to benefit patients have been clearly demonstrated. We anticipate that we may lose some patients – after all, they are infirm and 75 years plus. In a culture so often permeated with helplessness and despair it is encouraging to see that, through art therapy, there may be some hope of improving the quality of life for people in the agonising state of dementia and, moreover, that a major health care trust has sufficient confidence in our project to finance it.

Case vignette of an art therapy group with people with dementia

Finlay McInally

The art therapy group is made up of five members attending a social services day centre: three men and two women diagnosed as suffering from dementia. The group members were chosen randomly from twenty volunteers and so were not formally assessed for art therapy. The group consists of a co-therapist, a male care assistant from the centre and the following people:

- Arthur, who attended for part of the first session but quickly decided he didn't want to stay. He has made occasional contact since, usually at the beginning of a session.
- Oliver, who returned to the group after an unexpected three-week absence when he went with his wife for a stay at a respite home.
- Deirdre, whose husband has recently died. Prior to the session her care-worker informed me that the funeral was to be the following day, and that Deirdre has been 'a bit up and down'.
- Jack, who is the oldest member of the group and has found it difficult at times. The art work has reminded him of school and being a child. He has struggled with his deteriorating physical health and issues around dependence.
- Sylvia, who was quite artistic in the past, has seemed ambivalent and depressed within the group.

This was the seventh session of ten. We meet in a well-stocked art room for one hour. The room is private, and the centre staff respect the confidentiality of the group. Art work from previous sessions is to one side and there are drawing materials, paint, paper and clay set out on the table.

The group co-therapist collects the group members from the lounge. Deirdre arrives first and looks round the room as if in recognition. She rearranges some of the chairs haphazardly and wonders out loud what to do and where to sit. Jack enters the room, appearing frail and vulnerable. He sits heavily in a chair.

The co-therapist arrives with Sylvia. Deirdre, who has paired up with Sylvia in previous sessions, says she does not remember her. I say that we are still waiting for Oliver. There are moments of silence. I mention that there are two more sessions left before the group ends. There is more silence and a feeling of tension as they look round the room but not at each other. Sylvia looks up at the ceiling. Deirdre follows a fly with her eyes and then suddenly reaches for some clay on the table. We offer an assortment of paper or clay to the others. Sylvia accepts a small blue sheet of paper. Jack takes a sheet of white paper. He looks as if he is not sure what to do with it, and says, 'I can't do it.'

Oliver comes into the room. His wife hovers in the doorway and says 'Hello'. (I have previously discussed with her the confidentiality of the group and the art work.) Oliver looks depressed. The others barely acknowledge him and I introduce him to the group again. Deirdre now says she remembers being in the group before. I ask Oliver how it has been without the group for three weeks. He says he has not thought about it but that he knew the sessions lasted for ten weeks. He works on a clay racing car where he had left off, continuing a process of fixing the different parts of the car together.

Deirdre silently moulds a piece of clay, gently stroking, pulling and smoothing it. She looks determined and concentrated but seems sad and close to tears. Sylvia has chosen a blue pencil but seems reluctant to use it. She hums a tune and is accompanied by Deirdre whistling a different tune. There is a sense of them passing time and I am reminded of whistling in the dark to keep away frightening thoughts and feelings.

Sylvia: 'It's difficult to know what to do.'

Deirdre: 'Everything is the same.'

Sylvia draws a rainbow. She comments that a rainbow only comes out now and again. Jack sits between Oliver and the co-therapist and he seems smaller and less comfortable since Oliver has arrived. He thinks he can hear a baby cry and at the same time mentions it is his birthday soon. Jack then asks Paul (co-therapist) to show him what to do, and Paul responds by drawing a circle. Jack rejects this, pushing the drawing out of sight.

Meanwhile, Sylvia has asked Oliver about his racing car (see Figure 10.1) and he responds enthusiastically, indicating the cockpit and the chassis. The communication seems quite flirtatious. Sylvia tells him that there are only two weeks left. I ask Oliver if the car has a driver and he points him out to us.

There are ten minutes left of the session and Jack decides he wants to leave, turning to say goodbye to us.

Deirdre has been cutting a piece of clay in half and now attempts to fit the pieces back together. She says, 'I don't want him to go.' She comments that the clay 'ages at the same time as me'. This reminds me of her recent bereavement and I ask if the clay 'dies' at the same time as her, too. She says 'Yes!' loudly. She decides that the joined pieces of clay have become a dolphin (see Figure 10.3) and that it is now finished.

Sylvia's drawing of the rainbow seems more spontaneous and less hesitant than her previous images. She says, 'I'm getting better.'

Oliver finds it difficult to finish working on the racing car as the session comes to an end.

This session contains some of the themes of the group's development in the previous six sessions, as well as some of the members' concerns about the imminent ending of the group.

Despite the group members' difficulty with memory and communication, there is evidence to suggest that, at this stage in the life of the group, a certain cohesion exists. There are references to remembering the location and the faces, and to the group as a place in time. For example, Oliver mentions that the group will only last for ten weeks. Sylvia draws a rainbow that 'only comes out now and again'.

As in previous sessions, a strong theme of loss is apparent – loss of cognitive and physical ability, loss of relationships, of sexuality, role and identity. This theme is apparent in an initial sense of depression in the group's approach to the art. They feel bored, there's a feeling of avoidance and of 'whistling in the dark'. Jack seems to surrender altogether to his losses and the competition with Oliver, a younger group member. In previous weeks, Oliver's struggle to make a racing car has perhaps echoed his feelings of impotency. Deirdre separates and connects pieces of clay while talking about ageing and not wanting 'him to go'.

However, in exploring these feelings through the art-making process, which may hold memories of art from previous groups, there is the potential for reparation: pieces being fixed together, smoothed and stroked.

Stronger communication seems to develop through the working through of such feelings as loss, fear and helplessness. There are positive images: a rainbow, a dolphin and Oliver's racing car, now nearly complete and with a driver.

Notes

Full details of the methodology and results of this project, including the tabulated and statistical outcomes, are available in the report: *Evaluating the Use of Art Therapy for Older People with Dementia: A Control Group Trial* (Sheppard *et al.*, 1998), available from the Alzheimer's Society Brighton Branch, 206 Church Road, Hove BN3 2DJ, UK or from the editor. Further information concerning the current project, funded by PPP Health Care can be obtained from the editor: email diane.waller@virgin.net.

References

Beaujon-Couch, J. (1997) Behind the veil: mandala drawings by dementia patients, *Journal of the American Art Therapy Association* 14(3): 187–193.
Doric-Henry, L. (1997) Pottery as art therapy with elderly nursing home residents, *Journal of the American Art Therapy Association*, 14(3): 162–171.
Kahn-Denis, K.B. (1997) Art therapy with geriatric dementia clients, *Journal of the American Art Therapy Association*, 14(3): 194–199.
Sheppard, L., with Rusted, J., Waller, D. and McInally, F. (1998) *Evaluating the Use of Art Therapy for Older People with Dementia: A Control Group Trial.* Alzheimer's Society, Brighton Branch.

Shore, A. (1997) Promoting wisdom: the role of art therapy in geriatric settings, *Journal of the American Art Therapy Association* 14(3): 172–177.

Spaniol, S. (1997) Art therapy with older adults: challenging myths, building competence, *Journal of the American Art Therapy Association* 14(3): 158–160.

Yalom, I. (1983) *In-Patient Group Psychotherapy*. New York: Basic Books Inc., pp. 1–36.

Acknowledgement

Grateful thanks to Finlay McInally, Jenny Rusted and Linda Sheppard for their help in preparing this chapter.

Chapter 11

Changing the context of care: opening up the system

Interview with Kamal Beeharee

Diane Waller

Kamal Beeharee is the co-ordinator of services for early onset dementia in Brighton and Hove. A community psychiatric nurse, he is now manager of the Towner Club, which is a day club for younger people with dementia (normally under 65). The emphasis in the club is on freedom of choice and independence, and it offers a wide range of activities both within the building and in the community. It also offers a weekly art therapy group, which is discussed by Barry Falk in Chapter 9.

Kamal is very familiar with the services for elderly people with mental illnesses and dementia within the region. Through his training at the Tavistock Institute, he has strengthened his desire to create environments which are truly therapeutic.

We both felt that a conversation would best reflect Kamal's approach to his work, hence the interview.

D: Kamal, could I ask how you became involved in work with people with dementia?

K: I was working with people with learning disabilities, and then had the opportunity to work with older people with mental health problems in Brighton. I was transferred to a ward where there were a lot of people with dementia. From the beginning I had a special interest in learning more about dementia, because from that very early stage I felt it was not understood properly. People were not able to explain what was going on, they could not speak for themselves. I felt there was no one who spoke for them adequately. That was a very important motivation for me to work, to learn more, to feel more for people with dementia.

D: When you did your initial training, was it nursing?

K: It was mental health nursing. We only had very basic information about dementia. I did work on wards with people with dementia but I had little understanding of it. I was aware that people were depressed and anxious, that they had memory problems, but I couldn't really take these problems on board then.

D: I think perhaps public perception of dementia might have changed a bit – I remember that the thinking was, and probably still is, that it was something that happened to old people – called senile dementia – which had awful connotations – the thing that everybody dreaded – heads would be shaken – it was a very difficult, even taboo subject.

K: People were very misunderstood – people with dementia need to experience and use their abilities, or they get more angry, disappointed, frustrated and their problems get worse through the way we look after them. If we were to give them the opportunity to do more things for themselves, to use their abilities, they would feel more valued.

D: I think your position is that someone with dementia has cognitive difficulties but if we work on the capabilities as well as the deficits we can help them to relieve the frustration.

K: Very much so – people with dementia are very depressed at losing what they had; they need to use all their abilities. Their way of being is no different from anyone else's – they need to use their abilities to the full.

D: You said you had worked with people with learning difficulties (mental handicap), and the position of people with dementia reminds me of how people with mental handicap were viewed. It is very similar. I remember, in the 1970s, visiting a large institution which really upset and shocked me because it was dehumanising: people were graded, and I was horrified by that. They were in this old hospital, vegetating. Or going to so-called industrial therapy. The thing I remember most is they were making up those little packets of plastic cutlery for the airlines. At least the 'high grades' were . . . The notion that we just put people somewhere and leave them, just because they had a mental handicap, is terrifying. Mercifully things have changed quite a bit now. Did your experience of people with mental handicap carry over to people with dementia, your same attitudes – in that you are looking at them as complete persons with abilities rather than someone with just handicaps?

K: Yes. You have to look at the whole person. One of the problems is that people with dementia cannot express how they feel, their needs. You have to listen very carefully, at the cues they are giving, help them to understand the changes that are happening to them. The main problem is they have difficulty in expressing what they feel, and you really have to make an effort to understand. Then they are able to respond more, and life can be better.

D: When you began to specialise in this work, what was it like in terms of the organisation of services and the way that the hospital was managed?

K: People were categorised. At first I worked on an acute ward and there was one part where people with dementia were, and staff outside the ward took the view that it was not very glamorous work . . . I moved from the acute ward to the day hospital, then from there to a ward where most had dementia. I learned from people on the spot, not by going through academic exercises. I learned about dementia, and I realised that life could be made a lot easier for these patients if you try to understand them . . .

D: Did you get any support yourself there, as it sounds as if you were thrown in at the deep end?

K: Yes, I was, and it was only later on that I realised it more . . . but there was nobody at that time who specialised in dementia.

D: That's a very tough thing to have to do . . .

K: You had to justify yourself to professional colleagues. I had some support from my manager, not much understanding from colleagues. They looked down on that kind of work . . . The main problem was of resignation, on the staff's side. They were resigned, but there were people suffering, and *they* weren't resigned. It wasn't a life, sitting down doing nothing. It was non-purposeful . . . and the professionals were resigned for the people with dementia . . . thinking they were not capable of doing anything and just providing tender loving care. Staff were doing everything for the patients . . . people's individuality wasn't respected . . . all they needed was modification in the structure of daily life, and understanding. We are always modifying our lives, but people with dementia don't have as much power to do this. The staff were resigned, thinking 'this is downhill all the way' so they made sure the patients were not exposed to diseases, not taking risks, so that stops people from leading a full life.

D: That word 'resignation' . . . in my experience of visiting day centres the sense of resignation has been very strong on entering the building. People say things like, well, what can you do? Dementia – it's organic, so it will only get worse. It is a very heavy atmosphere, permeates the whole institution, and that I am sure attaches itself to the person with dementia, which is a vicious circle. The person with dementia gets depressed because they can't express themselves, so gets angry, then feels infantalised. The feeling of hopelessness reverberates among staff . . . everyone feels resigned.

K: There is an emphasis on protection, and it is overpowering . . . too much emphasis on safety is not just for the person, but against anything coming to the person. Protection, so much that people feel like they are in prison. It is usually staff protecting themselves. Why do we have to keep protecting people? Why can't they have a voice? Why do we have to decide for carers and people with dementia? They have to have a voice. The most important thing I felt had to happen on my ward was openness. You have to open all doors, I mean to allow carers to move in and out, people to express ideas and opinions. Otherwise it is very insular . . . the institution must change, it's a wall around you that must come down. It is part of the understanding of trying to break the barriers to understanding people with dementia . . . it's a question of breaking down the wall, of letting them come back into the world. Otherwise it becomes very much us and them. And that brings about a lot of unfair thinking which stops us enabling them to do things and to experience . . . At Towner Club that is what we are trying to do, allowing them to chose . . . there's openness and understanding.

D: It's a very radical philosophy, because if we think about the training of staff in mental health services we may say it is a bit better than it was in helping staff deal with the emotions that they have when working with severe mental illness or dementia. But still, the notion of being open is difficult for many people.

K: Very difficult, and unless you have a specialised unit for people with dementia you won't have openness, as there will be people with mental health problems who can express themselves and they will get the attention. Those who are not able to won't get it. It is very important to have the right environment, where their voices can get heard. Otherwise they will be frustrated. In the Towner Club they are not forced to do anything. They get frustrated, but have to learn how to modify their lives in order to survive . . . but generally they are *not* heard as to how these modifications can take place . . . and not helped.

D: It is as if they get blanked out . . . it's too painful to get in touch with the feelings . . .

K: All they get is physical care, washed, dressed, food, comfortable place to live . . . they are not outwardly suffering, but they must have a purpose in life . . . personally, I wouldn't be that bothered about the place I live in, that comes secondary, but the most important thing in life is to have something we enjoy doing. Lip service is paid, things are organised from one perspective, forgetting that simply sitting down in company, chatting, getting into their world, giving time, that is important.

D: It very rarely happens . . . The loss of the capacity to find words is terrible, you are living in a world where everyone else is communicating, you may have been a very articulate person, but you can't find the words . . . then being treated like an infant, doing silly games . . . that is the thing I found very depressing . . . the lumping together of everybody without attention to individual needs then provision of very banal activities, which is an insult to the intelligence of the people there. Why? 'Oh well they like to do it' . . . that is not my impression. I think the point you made is right, keeping at a distance, it does not threaten us.

K: We still have a long way to go in trying to see things from the point of view of the person with dementia and until that happens we shall have great difficulty in making life more comfortable for them.

D: When you were at Falconhurst[1] I know that you were trying to introduce a therapeutic culture, to change the ward into a therapeutic community.

K: Very much so. When we talk about a therapeutic culture, it was a culture which is normal: get up in morning, go down for a cup of coffee, instead of being tied down to an institutional regime.

D: The fact that it was a rambling building, I thought, was rather good, as people could go outside in the garden, or they could sit around, choose different places to sit, walk around the corridors safely, all those sort of things which I felt was good. I have some worries about purpose-built, smart new places . . . unless the attitudes change too . . .

K: When you come to think of it, most of the places we build are hospitals, but you don't need a clinical setting, you need a normal homely environment. I think that people with dementia are more at home in place like Falconhurst than in a very clinical setting, in hospitals where things are too medicalised . . . dementia is too medicalised . . . that is one of the big mistakes. We got away from that at Falconhurst. Talking about new buildings, even the contractors think in a medicalised way, and some buildings are more convenient for staff, people who are medically minded . . . I think you need a very homely place for people with dementia. But Falconhurst was overcrowded . . . it was not that the building was bad, it was the way that things were set up there that was bad, in the sense that it was overcrowded . . . but there is nothing better than a homely place, not a hospital, not like prison. Why don't we allow people the freedom to walk outside . . . why not have a place with grounds, nice garden, shops?

D: The environment where people are expected to live, it is so regimented . . . the worse place I saw was a ward in a local hospital which was so outrageous that I couldn't believe it . . . it had male and female dormitories at either end of the ward, which was on the top floor of an awful building, smelling of stale food. People were stuck there day after day, with nothing. Going out of the ward was impossible, due to the stairs. The ward manager had no idea what activities, if any, were provided. You would go crazy in such a place. That seemed to me one of the worst places I have seen, but I am sure there are many other places where people are incarcerated . . .

K: Most of the most beneficial provision for people with dementia originates from people who are not medically minded; for example, the Towner Club . . .

D: Say something about that, it's a good development . . .

K: It is a club; we want to raise awareness widely by sharing our ideas and findings. We are asking, how much can we enable people to express themselves, to participate – as I have said, I believe in openness . . . It is available for three days a week, two days in the day centre and one day we go out and see people, provide support, do one-to-one therapy, outreach in the community.

D: That is really new . . .

K: The operational policy says that on the Wednesday when we are not in the centre we go out and do interviews, identify the needs for one-to-one support, go to their homes when they have difficulty in going out, help people to feel able to go out, to get the confidence to go out. Teaching and reminding people of things they can do. We try and give practical support for the difficulties. Trying to keep a normal way of life. They are so overcome by their difficulties, their stress.

D: Keeping things as normal as possible is important for carers, for relatives, because it is very difficult to know how to manage the feelings you get seeing a loved one deteriorating in front of your eyes. There are such strong emotions, especially if the only alternative is for the person to go to a prison-like environment. It gives carers a shocking dilemma. I think this outreach work must be very important for the carers, too.

K: Very important. We take on if someone isn't well; if they can't access services, we inform people, help them to get what they need.

D: In my experience, as someone who works in the health care system, it was appalling being told, it is pretty hopeless . . . I had to fight to get what we needed . . . I was really struck by how difficult it was and it was a learning experience to be on the other side of such a barrage, to actually be in the position where you are rendered speechless yourself . . . your opinion doesn't count . . . but on the other hand there were many very kind and supportive people who were doing their best, genuinely wanted to help.

K: It's a question of politics. A lot of carers go through hell – professionals use politics to stop people accessing services or rather, denying their need, denying that people meet the criteria to access services. It happens a lot . . . even with CJD. There are professionals who feel that even many people don't meet the criteria for services, for long-term health care.

D: This tussle between health care and social services, it destroys innovative work; and the inability of services to come together has led to immense destruction. It is purely political – no one wants to spend money . . . the carer is in the middle of all this, with intense anxiety. Now, with the voluntary sector playing a part, this dismal situation is beginning to get attention. It is especially difficult because a lot of carers are elderly people, don't know how to get through the system, are at the mercy of events . . .

K: Certainly . . . and we do need specialist services, not one person who is overseeing things but a real team with specialised knowledge . . .

D: It seems as if the Towner is a good model, with the outreach etc., but I am conscious it is funded by charity.

K: By the national Alzheimer's Society, Brighton branch and Ardis, with some help from statutory services, but it is not a statutory service.

D: Extraordinary that all this pioneering work is being done all through charity . . . It is remarkable . . .

K: When I think about the trauma that sufferers go through, it deserves a better deal.

D: This work needs powerful voices behind it. Maybe it's difficult partly because nobody wants to imagine that they will have dementia, to contemplate such a thing. With drug addiction people can say they brought it on themselves – which isn't at all helpful to anyone, but with dementia nobody can say you chose it. I think it is such a fear that people want to keep away, don't want to get contaminated. There is more sympathetic presentation through the media now, but the profile through training has to be raised. I don't know many trainings in psychotherapy, for example, which address dementia in any depth.

K: I am trying to access some training; dementia counselling, it needs training, I need a place to learn more . . .

D: I am pretty sure that if you took the syllabuses of most of the counselling and psychotherapy training programmes you would not find any or much mention of dementia. Might find a cursory mention ... the attitude being, what's the point, how can you do psychotherapy with dementia patients? In art therapy we have always taken a different view. Art therapists traditionally worked with people who nobody else wanted to work with, and in the old days of chronically mentally ill people that was especially so. We acted in the belief that the individual is important, and there were some amazing outcomes, but it was not often taken seriously. I think we have a responsibility to try and ensure that training programmes address working with dementia.

K: A lot of people with dementia feel a stigma, so they deny they have it, but they have felt there is a stigma about the places where people are dumped.

D: I believe that this area (Brighton and Hove) might be better than many ...

K: One of the biggest problems we face is that there is not enough interaction with staff ... interaction is most important, promoting social interaction, it's a major thing but it so rarely happens, to sit down and spend a lot of time with people. Sometimes the people who are most trained spend the least time with the patients ...

D: I think your point about care getting too medicalised is true. Now we have Aricept, the wonder drug, I fear that people will say, now we have Aricept ...

K: It could be quite damaging in that carers could feel it is the answer, and forget about social interaction. It is no good just having medication. If that person has a good counsellor, social support, someone who understands, in other words a good team around, this is important.

D: The key is support for everybody, person, carer, team, and staff being able to tolerate feelings in themselves, not to run away. There are so many young carers, but they have no training. They go into the work very open, but they burn out very quickly as they don't have the capacity to deal with the emotions generated by a person with dementia. Personally I often got overwhelmed by Dan's moods – the rage, the frustration – and if you magnify this to a group of people feeling like this and not able to express it, it can be overpowering. In the art therapy groups we found that people were able to express rage, loss, and the pain at losing their role in life.

K: People must have a role, a purpose in life, and respect ...

D: Otherwise they become like a non-person, so what's the point ...

K: We have to ensure that institutions change, attitudes change ...

Note

1 Falconhurst was a residential NHS hospital for the elderly mentally ill, many of whom had dementia and/or additional psychiatric problems.

Chapter 12

Art as a therapy for Parkinson's

Nancy Tingey

How can people with Parkinson's paint?

'People with Parkinson's can't paint.' This dismissive remark, overheard as I was about to hold an art for Parkinson's class at a conference, is understandable. The most obvious symptom of Parkinson's is loss of controlled movement, manifested as tremor, contortion or inability to move at all. In this state how can anyone position anything accurately anywhere?

As one of my painting with Parkinson's group members observed, watching me move effortlessly to fetch something she needed: 'I used to be able to do that automatically like you.' Now she has Parkinson's she finds simple manoeuvres very difficult.

With Parkinson's the route for passing thoughts to the central nervous system has been impaired through lack of the chemical dopamine, essential to the smooth running of the track. Most of the cells which produce dopamine have been lost, or have died, for reasons which are not fully understood, and without dopamine the messages pass erratically, if at all, from one set of nerves to another. As a result, to the intense frustration of the person with Parkinson's, a perfectly reasonable 'instruction' from the brain is imperfectly transferred so that, for example, the intention to 'walk across the room and sit on that chair' may be interpreted through the central nervous system as 'do not move at all' or 'propel the body so fast it is unable to stop by the chair'.

To some extent the distressing symptoms can be relieved by medication and surgery. But there is still no cure and the disease is progressive. Understandably, anger, bitterness and depression develop as sufferers struggle to control their movements. And for younger people, or those who have led physically active lives, Parkinson's is particularly devastating. Diagnosis eventually leads to the end of life as they have known it.

Faced with a bleak future it may be of little comfort to recognise that in most cases the mental faculties of people with Parkinson's are unaffected by the condition. And, interestingly, their creative ability remains intact. Developing the premise that some of the mental processes considered essential to the realisation of imagination and originality are deficient in people with

Parkinson's, Professor Lakke, a Dutch neurologist, carried out a research project to assess levels of creativity in artists with Parkinson's before and after diagnosis. His assumption that creativity would be impaired by the progression of the disease proved not to be the case. Lakke discovered no 'impoverishment of originality or creativity' in artists who develop Parkinson's disease.[1]

Further, he found that 'artistic productivity remained amazing, despite considerable and limiting motor fluctuations', in the case of a sculptor who continued working after diagnosis,[2] and noted that the English author Mervyn Peake 'remained artistically productive despite very serious Parkinson-symptomatology'.[3]

Nine years after diagnosis John, an artist, wrote telling me he had been painting for thirty years when he was found to be suffering from Parkinson's 'but the disease had definitely not affected my desire to paint, or, fortunately, the ability to do so. In fact some of my friends tell me I have produced better work in recent years.'[4]

In trying to explain how a process as complex as creativity survives in parts of the brain and nervous systems known to be impaired by Parkinson's, Lakke suggests that autocuing, or using clues and triggers to initiate activity – a technique now commonly employed in the treatment of movement disorders – might in some way be circumventing the impaired motor programmes.[5]

The Movement Disorder Clinic in Melbourne, Australia and the Conductive Education Centre in Birmingham, England have been exploring this concept in depth, maintaining that people with Parkinson's who use the autocuing technique can do most things given the appropriate conditions, time and help.[6] They can even paint!

The clues in painting are the marks, made on the paper one at a time, each mark triggering another. Once the mark-making process is established it continues, providing there is no outside interruption, until the painting is finished. This process works most effectively when artists use their imagination, rather than a subject set before them, as inspiration. Listening to Melanie Brown, a facilitator at the Conductive Education Centre, I realised that the reason for this is that the intense interaction between artist and work surface is continually interrupted by looking up to refer to the subject. Drawing in this way is disconnecting for the person with Parkinson's. It seems that too many sequences are involved if the eyes have to leave the paper to look at something else and return. Concentrating directly on the paper does not present this problem. Conversely, there is no difficulty in, for example, drawing one's hand while keeping the pencil on the paper and not looking at the line. This exercise again involves a two-way concentration uninterrupted by a third sequence.

This phenomenon is borne out by the evidence of Suzanne, an artist who wrote to me, saying that since developing Parkinson's she found she tired quickly, especially while working from nature (still life, model or landscape), particularly feeling the strain when changing her focus from distance to proximity.

People with Parkinson's can paint with enjoyment if stressful aspects such as accurate drawing skills are played down. But how effective is art work in helping them cope with their condition? Wouldn't painting and drawing be similar to handwriting, which in Parkinson's becomes a tortuous activity as the disease progresses?

In trying to answer these questions I refer to the case of Keith, a professional engineer who also practised and taught calligraphy. Parkinson's forced him to retire early and give up his art work. 'My ordinary handwriting tailed off cruelly. Since taking my PD medication, however, I have found a great improvement in my calligraphic "hand", though not in my handwriting, and I have been able to potter with broad pens.[7] And while I have never found calligraphy in any way relaxing, I find my renewed activity provides exercises for my fingers, wrist and arm as well as some creative satisfaction. The process must use some other part of the brain, as well as finger muscles.'

Keith also found that as the letters became larger, involving the use of the wrist, then whole arm, as well as his fingers and thumb, the activity became more enjoyable, even intimating that 'making large short inscriptions in colours may be almost therapeutic'.[8]

Keith appears to be describing symptoms associated with so-called right- and left-brain thinking. 'Ordinary handwriting' is a stressful business as it involves thinking, organising and transposing words into symbols to make sense on paper, a demanding analytical process, whereas calligraphy is a creative activity in which the composition of shapes, lines and colours are as important as the meanings of the words. Rhythmic sweeping movements also appear to be beneficial, helping the nervous system run smoothly.

When we are experiencing difficulties with the left analytical side of the brain, do we make it easier for activities associated with the right side of the brain (for example, creativity) to take over? Neurologist Bruce L. Miller surmised, in relation to a disease called frontotemporal dementia, that when 'the left hemisphere was no longer inhibiting the visual hemisphere – the right hemisphere – so these visual activities were enhanced. It increased their interest in these artistic functions.' Also 'with the loss of their language functions, they were becoming more visually oriented'.[9] It therefore seems probable that as people with Parkinson's disease become less able to use spoken and written language to communicate their ability to use art to express themselves will increase.

Art as a therapy for Parkinson's

For art to become a healing process for Parkinson's the creative potential must be able to develop unimpeded by practical difficulties:

It is hard for any artist to work without encouragement and some support. People with disabilities may need physical help in setting up or preparing their materials. Yet it is these people especially who need an outlet for feelings that have no other form of expression. We do not need to be told what to create – indeed, who has the right to do that? But there may be real need for practical help and support for the adventure of creative work – to see that there is an uninterrupted time and enough space, and that the materials are always within reach and ready for use.[10]

So writes Rita Simon, who was eloquent in support of art groups for Parkinson's. In May 1988 Rita Simon had been the art therapist involved in a Parkinson's Disease Society holiday incorporating art and music therapy in which

a small group of people with Parkinson's Disease came together for two weeks to explore materials, such as paint, clay and creative writing as a form of self-therapy. Once they became familiar with the art materials, their imagination flowed and some fascinating and extremely expressive work was done. They were so absorbed that one could hear the proverbial pin drop. It was a joyful occasion for me to see the gallantry and liveliness that came for those facing serious disabilities, especially as my husband had recently found that he was also suffering from Parkinson's.[11]

Coincidentally my husband was diagnosed at about the same time that this was written, but it was not until late 1993 that I considered setting up an art group for people with Parkinson's. A year later Painting with Parkinson's began in Canberra, Australia with funding from a Special Needs grant provided by the local adult education centre.

As a practising artist with experience as an art educator and curator I ran the group initially as a recreational activity to help distract people from the trauma of having Parkinson's. It was only when a member joined Painting with Parkinson's on the recommendation of her doctor, who was concerned about her mental state, that I realised that without some art therapy training I would soon be out of my depth.

The award of a 1996 Churchill Fellowship enabled me to travel overseas for three months to develop my understanding of art as a therapy for people with Parkinson's disease, to learn strategies to help them find relief through art activities, and to gain information to encourage the establishment of appropriate art programmes throughout Australia.[12]

As it turned out I discovered only two centres which dealt specifically with art as a therapy for Parkinson's. These were in Italy and the USA, and the one in America hadn't actually begun a programme. I then looked at a number of other organisations and met individuals who were familiar with art as a therapy for other physical disabilities, next looking at other therapies and support groups for Parkinson's, the comparative values of art as therapy, and art therapy and psychotherapy in the treatment of illness – as well as the exhibition of work by people with disabilities. I studied programmes which made art in its widest sense available to people with disabilities – through day centres, hospital initiatives and art gallery education programmes.

I also followed up research on the creative process in relation to Parkinson's disease, and the work of artists who developed Parkinson's late in their careers, as well as poets and painters who used their art to express their feelings about Parkinson's after diagnosis.

In addition I examined practical issues such as strategic planning finance and funding, voluntary and paid staffing, acquisition and organisation of workspace, publicity and advertising, equipment and materials, exhibition and presentation of art work, and transport for people with disabilities.

It was the steepest learning curve of my life. And on my return to Australia in July 1996 I completely revamped Painting with Parkinson's.

Five experiences in particular had had a profound effect on my thinking. The first was time spent with Conquest, the Society for Art for Physically Handicapped People in Surrey, England. Ursula Hulme, founder and leading spirit, directs all her teaching efforts into encouraging creativity by releasing the subconscious, expressing emotions and allowing the imagination to flow. She introduced me to the power of doodling, an activity then expanded on by Rita Simon: 'Some artists need to start work each day by doodling freely to get the imaginative circulation going.'[13] Rita Simon also opened my mind regarding the meanings of art therapy versus art as therapy and psychotherapy. I realised that without years of further training art as therapy was my forte.

The third encounter which profoundly affected me was a visit to Midge Balkwill's yoga group for people with Parkinson's in Margate, England.[14] Those who had been practising yoga for an hour or more no longer wore the Parkinson's mask-like expression. They felt relaxed and refreshed.

I was wondering how to combine medication and art activities when I travelled to Milan to experience the Italian Parkinson Disease Association art programme. A trained art therapist whose husband, like mine, had Parkinson's disease, the co-ordinator Attilia Cossio, had devised a special curriculum inspired by the teachings of Rudolf Steiner, exploiting the therapeutic qualities of light and colour.[15]

Attilia Cossio explained: 'The process of painting is more important than the finished design. In this form of art therapy members express themselves through painting, enjoying the colour and meditating while painting.' She invited me to observe two of her classes, a new one in Milan and her original group in Monza which had been running for three years. (See Chapter 4 for elaboration of Cossio's work.)

Cossio worked on Rudolf Steiner's theory that the process of spreading paint in mist-like layers has a calming and therapeutic effort on the mind.

Because the paint cannot easily be controlled the opportunity to stimulate the imagination and draw on subconscious images is enhanced. Steiner also related particular colours to emotional states.

In the Monza class members were free to choose whatever they felt like painting, though several used images conjured up by the guided visualisation as a starting point. Again the room soon became quiet and the level of concentration profound. In all the resulting paintings the colours were clear and luminous.[16]

Martina Thomson, writing about experiencing colour, states that

> The Steiner-trained 'artistic therapist' . . . will consider [the influence of colour] central to his or her task . . . For me the colour blue, ultramarine, or rather a mixture of blues from ultramarine towards cobalt and light turquoise, has an infinitely satisfying effect. It is as though those colours make something reverberate within me or accord with it. Or, one might say, I have a need for the effect blue had on me.[17]

As blue is commonly believed to have a calming effect on the nervous system it may be particularly therapeutic for people with Parkinson's. Certainly all the groups I have observed using this colour appear to find it immensely satisfying.[18]

Later on in my Fellowship travels I came across a programme which used meditation to stimulate expressive use of colour in painting by people unaffected by Parkinson's.[19] This reminded me of research by Moya Cormick, a Jungian art therapist living in Australia, which compared coloured drawings made before and after following Manfred Clynes's sentic cycle meditation programme.[20] The later drawings were markedly more expressive than drawings made immediately before experiencing the cycle. When Moya Cormick developed Parkinson's she led a sentic cycle session for Painting with Parkinson's which affirmed her findings.

I also took part in a programme called CREATE (Center for Research Education, Artistic and Therapeutic Endeavors) at the Struthers Parkinson's Center in Minneapolis. CREATE embodies a holistic approach to the treatment of Parkinson's, combining medical facilities with complementary therapies. As I watched rhythmic movement in the relaxation exercise class, listened to a poet with Parkinson's relate his experience of painting to music, observed a speech therapy session and discussed with a research scientist how messages pass through the nervous system, the format of a Painting with Parkinson's programme addressing needs specific to people with Parkinson's began to take shape.

The Director of the Struthers Center, Ruth Hagestuen, defined art therapy as 'a process of presenting the opportunity for people to create and externalise images with the help of art materials'.[21] At the Center she emphasised the potential of creative expression to help sufferers come to terms with

Parkinson's disease. It was also clear that for people with Parkinson's to express themselves freely through their work, and to make the most of this to improve their quality of life, a holistic approach was needed.

As all the members of the Painting with Parkinson's group in Canberra also belonged to the local support group they were able to access information and other activities relating to Parkinson's. We ran yoga and t'ai chi courses, took groups to the exhibitions at the National Gallery, walked in the Botanic Gardens, and invited medical and complementary therapy speakers to monthly meetings. Some members sang; others read aloud the stories and poems they wrote. Over the next few years we drew on these resources and added to them to broaden the scope of Painting with Parkinson's.

One of the most moving innovations was a session with a sound therapist, Dian Booth, who brought along a magical range of Asian and African percussion instruments. For Painting with Parkinson's she played her violin while the group painted to the music. She then invited each member of the group to select an instrument from her collection and play it in front of the work they had just painted. As they played she improvised on her violin in accompaniment.

Later Dian rang melodic gongs as people painted, responding to the meditative atmosphere created by the sonorous chant which resonated through the room. Most extraordinary was the response of Jack, an intensely musical member of the group. Dian had invited anyone willing to play a rare, a sitar-like instrument she had brought along. Jack struggled to reach the instrument, 'freezing' with apprehension. Tentatively he began to pluck the strings. Over and over again he played the four lingering notes, gradually losing himself in the sounds. As he finished he rose and walked tall temporarily free of Parkinson's symptoms.

Following-up on this encounter we were fortunate to bring in music therapist Elisabeth Pillgrab in Canberra to work on a regular basis with the group. Although the healing power of music in the treatment of Parkinson's disease is well documented,[22] it was a revelation to see how Elisabeth used rhythmic tunes to encourage everyone to walk and dance. Even those who normally relied on walking frames found their feet. Soon everyone was singing and improvising on percussion instruments. Then Elisabeth played recordings – chants and ethereal pieces – to which everyone painted. Just as Lakke had found creativity unaffected by Parkinson's disease, so researchers Thant and McIntosh proved that the 'rhythmic entrainment mechanism remained intact'.[23] The combination of music and art therapy provides a ready recipe for healing, for which Elisabeth Pillgrab was the catalyst.

Other tutors working with Painting with Parkinson's combined clay sculpture with group poetry, ran marbling and silk painting sessions, and introduced the group to print making. Between us we constantly challenged them. While respecting Attilia Cossio's advice on limiting materials and methods so that variations in mental states could be clearly detected, we rang the changes to keep stimulating the mental capacities and nervous systems of people with Parkinson's.

If I noticed a painter's work becoming laboured or the technique unrewarding I would encourage them to try new materials and different ways of applying them. For instance, Norma became frustrated trying to draw with some graphite sticks which she had chosen. I suggested she might like to sample some new coloured inks by applying them to wet paper with droppers. The result was dramatic as Norma became totally engrossed, discarding the graphite to watch the brilliant ink colours merge and spread, carefully drawing lines with the tips of the droppers to link the pools of pigment.

In another Parkinson's group Mildred complained that holding a brush in her dominant right hand hurt her arm. For a while changing the brush to her non-dominant left hand solved the problem, but this was difficult to maintain as Mildred had Parkinson's dementia and the change of grip made her feel insecure and lose confidence. The action of applying liquid acrylics with droppers, however, employing the muscles of the dominant hand in a different way, caused no pain. Mildred enjoyed this new way of working so much that she began to interact with the group for the first time. Taking up this cue the whole group sang with her in the following week's session. Mildred again became animated. The change in her was extraordinary. She began signing her name instead of using the mark to which she had previously resorted.

Although wet-on-wet watercolour painting with brushes or fingers leads the field in techniques suitable for people with Parkinson's, the art tutor or therapist needs to be continually at the ready with alternatives in case a painter is experiencing trouble. Any kind of frustration will increase stress levels. And for people with Parkinson's, who are already unable to carry out many normal activities, adding painting problems can only be counterproductive. The process of making a mark, literally, for anyone with Parkinson's is so important that almost any means will justify the end. Unable to make the impression on society, which was their birthright, people with Parkinson's to some extent rediscover their belief in themselves when they make, for example, a mark on a piece of paper or an impression in a lump of clay.

While facilitating an art group in a nursing home I met Helen, the only participant with Parkinson's. Emotional and easily upset, Helen became agitated when she could not make her felt pen connect with a piece of paper on a board only inches away. With the help of a volunteer assistant we adjusted her wheelchair and raised the support with the paper until it touched the pen tip. As Helen watched marks appearing she relaxed and found she was able to draw confidently, making sweeping curved lines. Her demeanour changed to one of pure delight, an amazing transformation.

Unable to communicate, Betty sat immobile in her wheelchair at the day centre for hour after hour. However, when I gently held a pen between her fingers and moved a piece of paper to make contact, she stirred. Watching Betty's body language, to sense which way she wanted me to go, I slowly turned the paper so that she could draw an orange line all round the edge. Then she purposefully drew a second orange line just inside the first. She continued by placing a third line outside the first line and a fourth between the first two. When she indicated she was ready, I exchanged the pen in her hand with another. Betty then drew green lines across the rings, spacing them evenly all round the paper to make an image which looked rather like a railway. I can only guess at her intention, but it was clear that the process of making a mark was in itself enough to stimulate her sense of self. For the first time in months, so staff told me, Betty smiled.

Describing how painting had helped Jock through his last few years, his wife wrote:

> When my husband was diagnosed with PD several years ago, I became a full-time carer. I read books, listened to cassettes, attended seminars, hoping to find a way to help this emotional and physically limited man. It wasn't until he reluctantly agreed to 'try out' the Art for Parkinson's Group that I became aware of his need to find a way to express himself. Jock had been a professional soldier, used to commanding men. In the art group he 'told' the stories of his exciting life in colour on paper. Almost monosyllabic as dementia developed he became animated and lucid when talking about his paintings.[24]

Jock started painting in dark blues and browns but soon moved to reds and oranges. His later work became luminous with soft spots of pale pink and yellow. Jock's wife asked his psychologist about the changes. He explained that as Jock painted he became happier, and in turn his paintings reflected his contentment.

Jock communicated almost entirely through his painting. He appeared to live through it and it became his world. Gloria, on the other hand, was verbally articulate, using her painting to illustrate a poem she had taken an active part in composing with the group, titled 'This is Parkinson's My Friend':[25]

> 'I just found out
> I have Parkinson's'
> The group is what you need
> For where the Doctors fail
> They fail to understand
> the frustration, entrapment, depression
> life sentence, lethargy, dependence.
>
> Washing, walking, eating, shaving, cleaning,
> cooking, talking, writing, concentrating
> Now difficult

Drugs essential
but bring hallucinations, paranoia, dyskinesia

Swinging high to low
See-sawing out of balance

But feelings become acute
Compassion, empathy grows
The Group supports
The positive
The warmth
The friendship
The laughter
Parkinson's makes me anti-social

The Group shares interests, creates pictures
Music, sculptures, poetry,
cakes and tea
The Group relates to me, not my disease.

Another articulate member of the group, Belle, found it easier to tell the
story of her life through drawings than speaking directly to her audience. To
talk and maintain eye contact can be disconcerting at the best of times, but
for those with Parkinson's it is daunting. Art work, though, acts as an inter-
mediary, lessening the stress of confrontation as we study the art work rather
than the speaker. Belle had been a mathematics teacher with a sharp analytical mind. She took up painting after being diagnosed with Parkinson's as
she was keen to develop new interests. But she found making the first marks
difficult, questioning every move. Painting to music helped to relax her, as she
was intensely musical and could lose herself in the sounds. Belle also found
painting with her fingers stimulating. For her the combination of touch, sight
and sound were most rewarding. As Hagestuen says:

> Listening to music while finger painting can help calm tremors and dys-
> kinesia, release tension and pain and soothe a troubled spirit. It provides
> sensory stimulation as participants feel the paint on their fingers, see
> colour emerge on paper and hear the accompanying music . . . Multisen-
> sory art therapy allows people to work at their own pace and skill levels
> and build self-esteem as it brings more clarity to a person's identity. The
> more senses used during an activity, the greater the healing opportunity
> for mind, body and spirit to become integrated.[26]

Kick-starting movement

Although people with Parkinson's cope best with one activity at a time, if rhythm and touch or some kind of external instruction are brought in as part of the process these appear to aid rather than interfere with the action. In Andras Peto's conductive education programme, 'Activities were often accompanied by well-known poems and songs, the strong rhythm facilitating the action.'[27] Otherwise, when painters with Parkinson's want to brush marks on paper they may not be able to persuade their muscles to co-operate. As Melanie Brown at the National Institute of Conductive Education in Birmingham explains: 'You know what you want to do but your body can't do it without going through a programme.'[28]

If, however, a message comes from outside the body, through, for example, listening to a series of instructions, this circumvents the problem. This is one of the areas in which a skilled facilitator in a Parkinson's art class has an important role to play. For instance, in a sculpture session a series of prompts about kneading clay, flattening it, incising it with a tool and pressing fingers or objects into the clay, given one at a time, will usually produce appropriate responses. This does not mean that the tutor is making creative decisions on behalf of the student, such as deciding how thin the flattened clay should be, or what kind of marks should be made with the tool, but rather that s/he is giving objective guidelines to help the person with Parkinson's translate ideas into actions.

Other useful kick-starts are making marks in time to music, 'playing the piano' with finger paint, or playing 'pass the painting' – a game where everyone paints while music plays, then, when the music stops, passes the painting to the next person to work on, again while music plays. All the works move on in pauses between passages of music, either clockwise or anticlockwise. After a few moves the paintings become quite complex and the painters become reluctant to pass them on. At this stage the kick-start has completed its task and the painters retain the work before them to complete at will.

The advantage of this game is that, knowing marks will move on and become anonymous, the painters have no concerns about placing them correctly. The disadvantage is that losing ownership of marks can be disconcerting.

As the effectiveness of clueing and cueing may fade with use,[29] the art tutor or therapist may find they have to vary starting techniques from week to week. Unfamiliar ways of drawing, for instance, with eyes closed, using both hands at once, or using the non-dominant or Parkinson's-affected hand work well. Also, themes such as 'taking a line for a walk', or any form of doodling, help stimulate movement as well as creativity.

Ursula Hulme found doodling an invaluable tool when introducing new members to her Conquest classes. She found that 'doodling steadies the hand of patients with Parkinson's disease'.[30] And Hagestuen reiterates 'Persons with Parkinson's report that as they became engrossed in a particular creative endeavour, Parkinson's symptoms are often diminished. As they became totally focused, they achieved a meditative state.'[31] As the tremor in Parkinson's is a 'resting' one it will tend to die down anyway when the sufferer becomes busy doing something with their hands.

In a Parkinson's art class Norman observed that his left Parkinson's-affected hand shook when he was finger-painting with his right (non-affected) hand. When the left hand took over the finger-painting it stopped shaking. Norman also noticed that the shape made with his right hand dominated the shape made with his left. Another member of the class, Albert, pointed out that when drawing circles with both hands the Parkinson's-affected hand made smaller rings than the other. I found it touching to see how these artists could talk freely about signs of Parkinsonism in their work, as though detached from them.

Describing how his tremor settled when he was drawing in a Parkinson's art class Charles joked: 'When I am sketching I forget about the Parkinson's and the Parkinson's forgets about me.' Art therapist Wendy Maiorana elaborates on this phenomenon by referring to a comment made by Oliver Sacks on p. 202 in his 1973 book *Awakenings*: 'The patient ceases to feel the presence of illness and the absence of his illness and the full presence of the world.' Maiorana continues by saying she

> saw what seemed to me to be 'awakenings' each time [my client] Martin picked up a pastel and began to study the space relationships between the forms before him, or to grapple with colour relationships . . . He seemed alert, utterly focused on the outside world and the task at hand, rather than preoccupied with his body.[32]

In affirming the value of art as therapy for Parkinson's Rita Simon stresses the 'importance of being able to lose [oneself] in an exploration and enjoy the freedom of unlimited expression'.[33]

The friend of another painter with Parkinson's wrote to me that 'Two or three years after being diagnosed with PD [my friend] started painting and found it so engrossing she sometimes didn't want to stop. When having difficulty sleeping she found painting in the early hours comforting.'[34]

There seems to be an obsessive element about the way some people with Parkinson's take to art-making. The activity becomes all-consuming, possibly as a reaction to 'freezing' times when the body cannot do anything, let alone paint. Lakke found, for instance, in his study of artists with Parkinson's, 'that during the on-periods one worked more intensively in order to make up for the time lost'.[35] Perhaps this explains why work by people with Parkinson's often appears so moving. In any case, some artists rise to the occasion by responding positively to the constraints imposed by Parkinson's.

The observation is particularly relevant in the case of Paul, an ace formation flier forced to give up his exhilarating career when struck down with Parkinson's. He suffered dreadfully from violent dyskinesias which, alternating with freezing spells, incapacitated him for hours. But for short periods in the painting group, using his violent movements to effect, he was able to cover his paper with amazing rapidity, producing works of extraordinary passion.

Even a stubborn tremor can be used to advantage. Lakke notes that 'the tremor's energy facilitates hatching',[36] and records artists who 'made use of the tremor automatism for "easy" hatching'.[37] Cliff's experience in an early Painting with Parkinson's class illustrates this point. He had been struggling to depict the spiky flowers of a callistemon (bottlebrush plant) with a pencil. I suggested he might find pen and ink more rewarding. He found the change to his liking, saying 'This is easy; you just hold the pen and the tremor does the rest!' In the same group Charles and Albert developed highly distinctive styles with hatched lines, systematically covering large areas of paper as though obsessed by the process.

I was often fascinated by the intensity with which members of the Parkinson's group worked. Once the first marks had been made the artists seemed to become consumed by the process, often repeating movements as if to savour them as long as possible while the going was good. For instance, Bob would rework his wave patterns for over an hour at a time, totally absorbed in creating swelling seas, while Jock would rework a passage obsessively with different coloured oil pastels. Maiorana also describes her clients working this way with pastels 'seemingly compelled to go back and forth, back and forth, with tremulous scribbling motions.'[38]

Painting with Parkinson's

Most of the case histories I have described relate to members of Painting with Parkinson's. At the time of writing this art group has been meeting regularly on Friday mornings for six years in the Australian National Botanic Gardens, Canberra, at the Joseph Banks Building which is easily accessible to people with disabilities.

In the first year the programme attracted twelve members, six men and six women, of whom most had been diagnosed with Parkinson's for at least five years. My husband Bob, in his fifties, was the youngest member of the group; and the eldest was 80. Carers and helpers joined in the activities. Since its inception nearly thirty people have taken part in Painting with Parkinson's. Class sizes have varied from a handful to fifteen as no one was ever turned away. At times we considered running a second weekly class and we combined forces with the Multiple Sclerosis Society in Canberra for a while. But the core Parkinson's group became attached to their Friday meetings and these continue to be popular.

Fund-raising occupied many hours. Sponsors included Rotary and other local philanthropic organisations, as well as government, health and community education sources. Painting group members also supported their course with weekly contributions and participation in fund-raising projects. I felt from the beginning that it was important to offer the best working conditions we could afford in order to show that Painting with Parkinson's was a serious venture. People with disabilities are entitled to the same high standards which the rest of the community expects.

To this end the tutors and therapists were always paid standard fees to run sessions. And the best-quality materials were used, including fine liquid watercolours and paper from the suppliers of Steiner schools. Other materials were bought from school supply stores and art shops. Tools such as brushes, oil pastels and felt pens (which had thick shafts making them easy to hold) were chosen, as well as clear, brightly coloured paints and inks or liquid acrylics which were attractive to use and non-toxic. Clay was provided by the tutor responsible for the activity, as were materials for specialist sessions such as silk painting or marbling.

Volunteer helpers took care of art materials and refreshments. Painting with Parkinson's was a large group to manage so volunteers were essential and treasured assets. Sometimes there would be two tutors or therapists working together (for example in a combined music and painting session) or in adjoining rooms when sculpture or clay work was offered as well as painting. On these occasions there would often be five or six volunteers helping.

By trial and error we found that the most appropriate facilitators were either therapists or art teachers used to working with adults and people with disabilities in an art school setting. These were most likely to understand the value of mark-making and 'going with the flow' rather than drawing from life. When the time came for me to move on I was therefore fortunate to be able to hand the group over to a printmaker who worked in this way himself and had established a reputation for inspiring his students to develop their creative abilities with the simplest and most accessible techniques.

It is difficult for the unskilled printmaker to predict exactly what will happen to an image during the printing process. Sensitively handled, the image will be enriched, acquiring texture and tonal range barely anticipated in the original mark-making activity. As with wet-on-wet watercolour, painting control of the process is taken out of the artist's hands and transferred to the whim of the materials.

As people with Parkinson's normally struggle to control every aspect of their lives, permission to relinquish being in charge relieves this stress. It is a gift to be allowed to respond to the process as it unfolds instead of having to go through the daunting prospect of controlling outcomes. Art for Parkinson's allows the unpredictable to be revealed in unexpected ways within a secure and caring environment. The following poem describing this sheltered workshop was written by the counsellor for Painting with Parkinson's:

This is Painting with Parkinson's

She lives alone
Is determined about her independence
Drives
but risks only familiar tracks now

She arrives at class flustered, frustrated,
even angry today:
A visit to the doctor this morning
with new symptoms
but little sympathy or support returned

She could've gone home
but the care brings her to class.
She frets about herself, experts, driving home . . .
Her first painting of trees,
bold and angry red
emotions flowing through the brush.

Her second
a calming green
with subtle shades of sky
and suggested hills.

Her load lighter now.

She calls us her family;
a community
of giving and receiving

The agendas are many:
support,
acceptance,
belonging, creating,
caring and cared for
mixing

A place where souls are nourished
and restored
This is Painting-with-Parkinson's.

Marjorie Crombie, 13 November 1998

Two issues arising from this introduction to Art for Parkinson's are explored here in more depth. One is the fear of failure, the other the role of discussion and evaluation.

Fear of failure is an all-too-familiar sensation for people with Parkinson's, so it is critical that the art activity be an enriching and liberating experience from the beginning. When a participant in an art group has a disappointing experience it is often because the environment has been unsettling or disruptive, the facilitator has mismanaged the provision of materials at the appropriate time, or the participant has come to the session with a set preconceived idea about what they want to achieve – in a sense setting goals.

Conductive educators insist that it is counter-productive for people with Parkinson's to start with a goal in carrying out any activity. This means that, following through the example mentioned at the beginning of this chapter, an intention to 'walk across the room and sit on that chair' is likely to be carried out successfully by resorting to strategies which circumvent the nervous system. By concentrating on the processes involved in walking across the room, such as lifting and lowering the feet and spacing the steps one by one, preferably while counting out loud or listening to relevant instructions, the body can be persuaded to start the process. Reaching the goal as a by-product comes as a surprise!

This principle can be applied to art as a therapy for Parkinson's by following the experience of Ann, a painter who enjoyed many art activities, but was constantly disappointed by her efforts to paint scenes she had conjured up in her mind before she arrived at the class. On the other hand she found painting to music satisfying and loved the exercise of 'taking a line for a walk', discovering the shape of shoes among the meanderings. She also enjoyed tearing and layering coloured tissue paper at random in collage work.

Eventually she realised that the more determined she was to achieve a set outcome the more likely she was to find the task beyond her, at the same time missing out on the creative 'accidents' along the way which might have opened up new paths of discovery for her. It is important for participants to allow the process to take its course. There can be no failure if everyone responds freely and honestly to the stimuli they experience while art-making.

Discussion and evaluation

In running the discussion part of the programme I was aware that most of those involved were wary of analysis and self-evaluation. They had joined the group for social reasons and to take up a new activity to replace those they could do no longer. Discussions about their work sometimes touched on emotional issues, but more often centred on the ways in which the art activity triggered memories, provoked tactile sensations or caused physical relief from Parkinson's symptoms.

To some extent this situation arose because none of the facilitators was fully trained in psychotherapy and group dynamics. As Diane Waller suggests, 'Without the confidence that a thorough training and experience in group dynamics should impart, art therapists were probably wise to try and "keep the lid on".'[39] However, I kept detailed notes about each member of the Painting with Parkinson's group and photographed most of their work in case the opportunity arose for further study by more appropriately qualified therapists.

The following more general observations have been taken from my report on the Art for Parkinson's pilot trial sponsored by the Parkinson's Disease Society in England in the year 2000:

> One of the volunteers observed that when the class started members were very self-conscious and aware of how others work but by the seventh week they didn't seem to mind what others thought about them.
>
> At least two members of the group were sceptical about the course but changed their minds as they became involved in the creative process and surprised themselves with what they achieved. One was angry to start with but her mood gradually changed.
>
> One carer said she 'gets away from it all in the class' but also found that participating in the art group led to her being interested in watching art programmes on TV. Other members said they looked at things around differently after learning to paint.

For one member at the group who has Parkinson's the outcome was so remarkable it is worth describing in more detail:

> Fred hardly spoke in the first sessions but by the end was contributing to discussions like everybody else. His wife and daughter said the change in him was extraordinary. Before diagnosis Fred had many interests and was always doing something. As Parkinson's developed he became anti-social and disinclined to do anything. However on the morning of the third class Fred rose early, unaided, dressed himself including pulling on his socks and fastening his buttons and declared he was ready to go, well before time. Not only was he keen to paint and draw, he renewed his interest in other aspects of his life, including taking up driving again, and became sociable.

Artists with Parkinson's

As noted in the comments on the pilot trial, occasionally someone joins a Parkinson's art group to renew their role as a practising artist. They approach the group activities from a challenging perspective, already having high expectations of their abilities. This may make it difficult for them to come to terms with the changes which Parkinson's disease has caused in their way of working. But if the artists are able to adapt to the changes, and try different materials and techniques, they may still gain satisfaction from their work.

Where the artists allow themselves to use their art as a vehicle for self-expression, baring their souls as it were, they can experience the same feeling of release as group members who respond more directly to the programme, having no preconceptions about their abilities. In support of this observation I offer the case histories of Sheila and Jack. Sheila was an eminent potter who made highly polished figure studies in clay until she was forced to stop work because she lost strength in her arms when Parkinson's developed. At first, in the art group, she tended to worry about her painting technique, being concerned about the rough finish and her lack of control. Then she began painting moody romantic landscapes with wet-on-wet watercolour, often using her fingers to apply the paint. When she discovered monotypes – taking prints from paintings she made on the table top – she developed an expressive, highly charged emotional style which brought her intense relief. Overall Sheila found that the combination of relaxing environment, music and painting or drawing encouraged her to think creatively, becoming more responsive to her surroundings and less obsessed by her illness.

Jack enjoyed painting coastal landscapes, flowers and portraits in pastels, attending classes at the local art school until his Parkinson's symptoms made him feel too conspicuous to continue. When Painting with Parkinson's began Jack was the first to realise the advantages of joining a sheltered workshop. It soon became clear, however, that his pastel painting now smudged easily and frustrated him. I suggested a change of direction, offering him pens and brushes and coloured inks. He took up the challenge enthusiastically, painting glorious fantasies to music and recording colourful memories of his favourite haunts. Jack also painted to express his horror of tragic events. Painting sustained Jack until the day he died of heart failure in his late seventies. In the last weeks of his life, when he could no longer attend classes he would paint at home or in hospital, wheelchair-bound and on oxygen. Painting became his *raison d'être*.

Jack used to maintain that the beneficial effects of painting in the Parkinson's art group would last up to two weeks after a session. Few members recorded such a strong response, but in general participation in art classes for Parkinson's was shown to have relieved depression and to have increased self-esteem. Some members also recorded becoming more confident and taking pride in their work. Others said they became so absorbed in the process that they forgot abut their problems. Finding the experience both stimulating and calming at the same time was often noted, as were social factors such as the opportunity to make friends. The empathy and accepting attitude of the tutors, therapists and helpers were also mentioned.

Although most of this information was gleaned from discussions with group members or comments they made on evaluation forms and questionnaires, the most telling revelations came from their art work. In a letter of support to a funding body in 1998, printmaker John Pratt summarised Painting with Parkinson's as

> a context where the participants gain considerable emotional and physical release through a range of activities including painting, printmaking

and sculpture. The imagery is intrinsically rich and expressive and of a testament not only to the inherent power of art therapy but also represents a significant contribution to the wider arts community.

Notes

1 Johannes P.W.F. Lakke, Art and Parkinson's disease. Paper delivered to the EPDA (European Parkinson's Disease Association) General Assembly, held in Glasgow, September 1994. Also in conversation with Nancy Tingey in May 1996.
2 Lakke, J.P.W.F. (1999) Art and Parkinson's disease, in *Parkinson's Disease: Advances in Neurology*, Vol. 80 (edited by Gerald M. Stern). Philadelphia: Lippincott Williams & Wilkins, pp. 472–474.
3 Lakke, op. cit., 1994 and 1996.
4 Letter to Nancy Tingey, dated 1 February 1999.
5 Lakke, op. cit., 1999, p. 471.
6 For example, at the Movement Disorder Clinic Kingston Centre, Wattigal Road, Cheltenham, Victoria 3192, Australia and the National Institute of Conductive Education, Cannon Hill House, Russell Road, Moseley, Birmingham B13 8RD, UK.
7 Further research on the relationship between Parkinson's medication and creativity needs to be undertaken before conclusions can be reached on this topic.
8 Letter to Nancy Tingey, dated 23 January 1996.
9 Report by Rob Stein in the *Washington Post*, Monday, 26 October 1998.
10 *Parkinson's Newsletter*, December 1991, p. 19.
11 Ibid.
12 Nancy Tingey, Art as a Therapy for Parkinson's Disease. Churchill Fellowship Report 1996–7 (unpublished).
13 *Parkinson's Newsletter*, op. cit., p. 19.
14 Midge Balkwill was secretary of the Parkinson's Disease Society, Thanet Branch. Following my visit in 1996 Midge launched a new art group which, two years later, held an exhibition titled 'Against All Odds' at The Cliftonville Library.
15 Attilia Cossio, Il colore, la leggerezza e la malattia di Parkinson, 1995. Paper written for the first exhibition of work in Monza by the Italian art therapy group.
16 Tingey, op. cit., 1996–7, pp. 19–21.
17 Thomson, M. (1989) *On Art and Therapy, An Exploration*. London: Virago Press, 1989, pp. 75–78.
18 Attilia Cossio's group in Milan, April 1996; Painting with Parkinson's, Canberra, July 1996; Art for Parkinson's, Shrewsbury, May 2000. The blue oval exercise was also practised in art workshops at the YAPP&RS (Young Onset Parkinson's, Partners and Relatives) conference in Peterborough, June 2000.
19 Jenny Walter's 'Creative Painting' workshops, Crooklands, Cumbria, UK.
20 Neuroscientist Dr Manfred Clynes developed the concept of sentic cycles in which an audiotape is used to enable the safe release of negative, then positive, emotions.
21 Ruth Hagestuen, Parkinson Report, National Parkinson Foundation, USA, Spring 1999, p. 27.
22 M.H. Thant and G.C. McIntosh, New Music Therapy Research Studies. The effect of rhythm and music on the walking ability in PD patients. Paper delivered to the Fourth International Congress of Movement Disorders, Vienna, June 1996.
23 Ibid.
24 Letter of support for funding application, to Nancy Tingey, December 1998.
25 Poem written by the Canberra Painting with Parkinson's group co-ordinated by Peter Latona, September 1997.

26 Hagestuen, op. cit., p. 27.
27 Veronica Nanton and Andrew Sutton, Conductive Education: a Psychopedagogic Paradigm for Intervention in Parkinson's Disease. *Parkinson Magazine* (European Parkinson's Disease Association), Autumn 1996, No.7, pp. 7–12.
28 In conversation with Nancy Tingey, June 2000.
29 Veronica Nanton, Verbal Regulation, Conductive Education and Parkinson's Disease, 1984.
30 Used on a poster advertising Conquest classes. Conquest Art Centre, Cox Lane Day Centre, Cox Lane, West Ewell, Surrey KT19 9PL, UK.
31 Hagestuen, op. cit., p. 27.
32 Maiorana, W. (1989) When art is all there is: art therapy in the treatment of a man with Parkinson's disease, *The American Journal of Art Therapy* 28: 22.
33 *Parkinson's Newsletter*, op. cit., p. 19.
34 Letter to Nancy Tingey, 1996.
35 Lakke, op. cit., 1994.
36 Lakke, op. cit., 1999, p. 475.
37 Lakke, op. cit., 1994.
38 Maiorana, op. cit., p. 22.
39 Waller, D.E. (1993) *Group Interactive Art Therapy*, London: Routledge, p. 14.

Chapter 13

Circles of the mind
The use of therapeutic circle dance with older people with dementia[1]

Dorothy Jerrome

Introduction

This chapter describes the effects of using a form of community dance with older people with mental health needs. Some were in permanent or respite residential care, others were brought to a day centre by mini-bus from their homes. Most had dementia, a few were chronically depressed or had schizophrenia. The work described here covers a number of years, starting with some exploratory dance sessions in 1996. Most of the work took place in local authority day centres, though some involved private residential establishments.

The initial sessions convinced me of the value of the work, and a formal evaluation was designed involving a second series of dance sessions. The third phase involved broadening the original approach to include more chair-based dance and movement adapted to the needs of frailer participants. Currently the focus is on training issues, and the final part of the chapter offers guidelines for would-be facilitators of therapeutic circle dance sessions.

The nature of dementia

Dementia is a progressive and irreversible brain disease which gradually erodes the capacity to reason, to think, to learn and to remember. Some skills survive longer than others, however. The capacity to respond to music lasts almost to the end. People with dementia retain powerful feelings long after they have lost the capacity to express them through language. Relatives and professional caregivers sometimes prefer to think the sufferer is 'no longer there', and the once-loved person has somehow departed from the frail physical container (Gubrium, 1986). This possibility allows us to concentrate on caring for the physical body that remains. But an increasingly popular view is that it is not the mind that is destroyed by the disease but the capacity to express it (Goldsmith, 1996). The person with dementia is someone whose illness gets in the way of communication. The apparent 'slipping away' reflects a process of withdrawal to an inner world, 'some interior mindscape known only to herself'. But access to the emotional world of the person with dementia goes on being possible almost to the end if we are resourceful enough, and can bear the tragedy of such an ending (Sinason, 1992; Killick, 1994).

In the early stages of the illness there is a sense of loss which produces sadness and distress, and a vague awareness that something is wrong. The person with dementia typically experiences anguish, anger, denial, depression and eventually acceptance (Keady, 1997). Some people may never complete this process and stay permanently locked into a state of denial and anger. For them it is always 'other people' who are responsible for the loss of belongings or who have muddled their lives (Mills, 1998). Successful adaptation to the dementing process is a central theme in the writings of Tom Kitwood. He explores the relationship between the experiential or feeling self and the adaptive self which is formed through our social interactions with others. Dementia removes the cognitive supports that surround the adapted self and leaves the experiential self exposed and vulnerable. The experiential self is often immature or underdeveloped, and sometimes wounded by adverse early experiences. It is the part of ourselves we generally keep hidden and protected. We can begin to see that the person with dementia, incapable of pretence and exposing her undisguised feelings, is in a sense showing her true self. In this view, older people with dementia often exist in a state of greater emotional authenticity than those who care for them. Just as babies are extremely emotional beings with immature cognitive processes, so in dementia the emotional processes have more durability than the cognitive (Mills, 1998).

As the illness progresses, the need for reassurance in an unrecognisable world comes from distant memories of parent figures who once allayed fears and provided security through holding with arms and bodies. Our understanding of this process owes much to the work of Bere Miesen, a Dutch psychogerontologist, whose own interventions with nursing home residents are framed by attachment theory. His writings provided the inspiration for the Attachment Awareness and Dementia Care project in Hampshire (Mills et al., 1999) and informed the work described in this article.

Attachment theory shows us how the individual, by nature, is driven to form emotional ties with special persons – parents but also others. Attachment behaviour includes actions which try to achieve and maintain closeness. Attachment behaviour is activated in certain circumstances such as unfamiliar situations and the presence of fear, especially when one is alone. The theory also provides insight into how an individual might react to loss. Concrete attachment behaviour is strongest in the early stages of dementia, in relation to living relatives and carers. It takes the form of touching and turning towards, crying, following with one's eyes, and calling after. As the disease progresses this behaviour is replaced by what Miesen (1992) calls parent

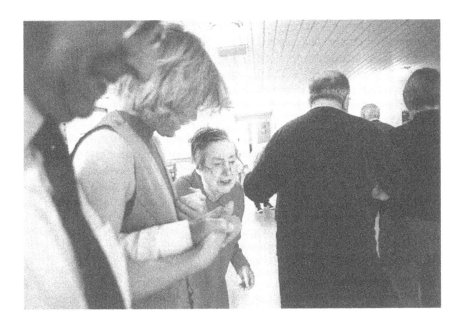

fixation. Calling on and referring to parents indicates that the need for safety is being met from within the person him or herself. Sooner or later, elderly demented persons think that their long-since deceased parents are still alive and they ask, for example, to 'go home'. Their perpetual requests for their parents or other long-departed attachment figures can be interpreted as a cry of distress, as a cry for security, rather than as a muted memory from the faded past.

In these circumstances, caregivers need to help the person with dementia to accept and explore the painful experience of loss and disintegration. The traditional approach to this task – reality orientation, which might involve 'correcting' factual inaccuracies – is being superseded by a new emphasis on processing emotions. Caregivers need to be attentive and active listeners, aware of verbal and non-verbal communication, and able to communicate empathy through positive body posture (Mills, 1998). The capacity of caregivers to communicate acceptance and love through touch helps to preserve a sense of self. This kind of touch can also alleviate problem behaviours like aggression and shouting, which are expressions of rage, frustration and despair (Stokes, 1996). In this personal environment the sufferer of dementia is free to be him or herself, with the help and support of others. This empowerment of a person with failing cognitive processes restores personhood, integrity, and a sense of the individual uniqueness of being (Kitwood, 1997a).

This account of dementia helps us to see why circle dance might make a difference in the lives of sufferers. It is a way of communicating through touch and rhythm. The circling and holding, the rocking and gentle repetitive movements, communicate acceptance directly and without words in the manner of early attachment experiences. The music touches something deep within the person.

As I write that sentence a powerful image comes to mind. Two profoundly ill people are emerging from the doorway to the residential unit. Largely lacking in speech and with poor co-ordination, but able to walk, they come straight towards the circle of dancers. Drawn by the music and waiting figures they move like sleepwalkers, apparently oblivious to other people. The circle parts for Beatrice (not her real name) and she passes to the centre, stopping for a moment as if in thought. Then she moves on and away to some unknown destination. As Leo reaches us his hands are taken by two young male care assistants and he starts to dance.

Dance at the day centre

In 1996 I started circle dancing at a social services department day centre in a specialist unit for older people with mental health problems. The observations which follow were produced after thirteen sessions. Each session lasted an hour, during which we danced about eight dances. The dances came from around the world: Russia, Greece, Israel, France, the Andes, the Balkan countries, and from Celtic traditions. The dance steps were adapted for this group – walks, sways, slip-steps, rocking – with much simplified rhythms. At first it was a case of trial and error. I learnt that it was best to hold hands, to minimise the risk of people wandering off in the wrong direction, and to dance in circles facing the centre so that we could see each other. Dances involving progression and facing in the line of dance were harder to control, as the dancers could only see the shoulders in front of them, and people stopped moving so that we all piled into one another. For the circle to progress to the right or left the presence of one or two care staff or older people who could dance reasonably well was essential. To assist with balance and to communicate the rhythm to the more impaired people I tended to use a close arm hold (locking elbows). A shoulder hold in the Greek dances had the same effect. Some of my notes, made after the sessions, give a sense of the experience:

> The session starts with a dozen or so old people assembling and sitting down round the edges of the fine wooden dance floor. I put on a tape and dance a bit myself before inviting them to join in. The women clutch their handbags – repositories of the self – and need to be gently parted from them. Sometimes someone like Angela, who used to be an opera singer, starts to improvise and we build her steps into a dance. It seems important to affirm her creativity and control over what is happening. Those in

the early stages of the illness like Jane are relaxed and happy here, glad to be able to do something well for a change.

Daniel has poor co-ordination and hardly moves. He has largely lost control over his muscles and his mouth hangs open, but he can smile and his eyes shine. Another very impaired person, Christine, with a blank, mask-like face and staring eyes, seems cross at first and says she is not staying. But she recognises and responds to the beauty and grace of the music, coming very close to tell me so. In a simple Breton dance, with a close arm hold and minimal movement, she starts to tell me about her work with deaf children. Colin is a 'ladies' man' and still flirtatious. He longs to join us – he used to do a lot of ballroom dancing – but his perceptual skills are poor and he cannot keep in the circle, drifting into the middle so that others cannot see. A care worker dances with him outside the circle and he is happy for a minute or two.

May is schizophrenic and hostile. In the first week she prowls around the circle talking angrily to herself, but at the end I see that she is dancing alone. The following week she joins in, but as we lift our feet (side close side lift) she kicks out, in time to the music! In week three I notice that she is wearing lipstick and beautiful gold dancing shoes; but her arms are rigid with tension. In week four she is missing – and I miss her. Since then she has appeared sporadically and dances from time to time. Her concentration is limited and she tires easily. Recently she has been calling me mother and addressing herself as May. She talks of her travelling days and sadness about the loss of her mother. Clara is also schizophrenic, with the palour of someone institutionalised for many years until her long-stay psychiatric unit was shut recently. She demands to know what I am writing in my notebook. My explanation that I need to record her name so that I do not forget it seems to satisfy her. She feels safest sitting down and looks on while we dance. The 'approach–avoid' style of May and Clara is consistent with the needs of many people with schizophrenia to limit or regulate emotional and social contact.

These were a few of the dozen or so old people who danced regularly. They represented a range of abilities, reflected in their use of language. Their verbal communications – greetings, thanks, reminiscences – ranged from conventional expressions like 'This is delightful, thank you so much, do come again!', and 'My sisters and I used to dance in the garden', to the words and phrases of time-disordered and aphasic individuals: 'Oh nice, isn't it a nice . . . nice music!' (with triumph as recognition dawns) and 'Mother [should be] here to watch me . . .'

It was a challenging group. Continuity was an issue, for they were often unwell and the weather affected their moods and energy levels. Some people were very volatile, suddenly becoming cross or fearful. At first I was tempted to 'jolly them along', as the staff were inclined to do. Levels of impairment like this are hard to accept. In an early session I became aware of the workers noisily counting time as we danced. I found myself joining in, and the counting went on with increasing intensity. Then I noticed that a group of managers was watching us from a doorway. The staff had been performing for them. The atmosphere at that moment was far from the kind of happy calm which I had been striving for.

I gathered from staff that the dance was helping to improve motor skills, balance and social skills. The circle was a social situation. The dancers made reference to each other, to the non-dancers sitting watching, and to the shared dances as pleasurable or too long or boring. Conversations went on between people dancing side by side. 'I used to do this at school you know'; other such personal statements were communications about the self, stimulated by the dance experience. Some encounters were very moving, as when Edward persuaded Mary to join the circle. Newly arrived for respite care, Mary was shy and nervous, refusing all invitations to dance. Edward, a gentle and courteous man at an advanced stage of the disease, offered his hand and waited until Mary rose to her feet. Kissing her on the cheek he told her, 'You are a lovely girl!' with a tenderness and respect perhaps once reserved for his wife or daughter. The rest of the dancers were delighted and made clear their own pleasure at Mary's inclusion in the group. In this way even intimate dyadic communications are made public and affirmed by others present.

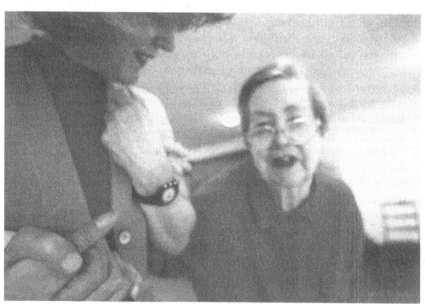

Circle dance as a learning experience

The staff also enjoyed the event. Their manager told me that there had been an increase in their involvement and interest in the clients who dance. However, dancing with clients is itself a skilled performance. While concentrating on the dance and helping people either side to move in time to the music, the staff also needed to attend to feelings. People's anxiety levels and concentration are affected by environmental factors such as the time of day and expected time of departure. In the afternoon sessions people were anticipating the journey home. Questions about transport, like the concern over handbags, are often about loss, anxiety and fear. The challenge of looking out for and addressing these feelings needs to be recognised. Work with this client group calls for an awareness of metaphor, and the personal meanings buried in words which no longer make sense. Unfortunately the work attracts staff whose powers of interpretation are sometimes limited. Leo, mentioned earlier, was standing next to a temporary care assistant who had a limited command of English (her native tongue was Japanese). During the round of introductions he struggled to ask her where she had come from. With enormous effort he found some of the words and tried to communicate but without success. Although several people in the end were asking Leo's question for him, the young woman continued to gaze at him blankly. It was a sad reminder that people like Leo deserve the highest quality of care but often do not get it.

When working in this way we need to be ready for all eventualities. On an afternoon session when people were worrying about getting away, and asking when the coach driver would arrive, Leo seemed to have worries of his own. He was unable to settle, anxious first that we move to the proper end of the room (we were in the carpeted area rather than on the wooden dance floor) and then that we wait until 'the musicians' had arrived. As I struggled to make sense of his words, he repeated 'Where is the music driver?' As I carefully addressed his apparent confusion, he added with a chuckle, 'It's a joke!'

The use of language in the course of the session was significant. Although dance offers a chance to communicate without words, there was actually a lot of talking at these sessions. Bright (1992) also suggests that dance stimulates language use, despite the location of linguistic skill in the opposite side of the brain from musical responses. We underestimate the capacity of people with dementia for speech. The creative use of language has been noted by Killick too: 'The speech of many people with dementia is unusually creative – it exploits the full range of linguistic possibilities, with particular emphasis on new combinations of words, sound patterns and figures of speech' (Killick, 1998: 92).

Early questions prompted by the dance experience were about what to expect from this group and how best to work with them. Should I be playing music which matched their moods, however dark, to allow them expression, or should I be choosing happy music to cheer them up? Like Bright (1992) I was inclined to think that music allows feelings of anger or depression to come to the surface but does not cause them. Above all it was important not to use such activities as dance defensively, to deny the pain and loss of dementia (Sinason, 1992; Terry, 1997).

How would the dancers remember me and the steps from session to session, when their short-term memories were so impaired? I was told that they could learn experientially if they were emotionally engaged and enjoyed the learning experience. In conventional music therapy, the musician uses old and well-established memory traces dating back to childhood and early adult life (Bright, 1992). But unlike the popular songs of the pre-war era favoured by activities co-ordinators, international folk dance is generally unfamiliar to people with dementia. However, it draws on early memories of rhythm and movement.

How important was it to get the steps right? Compared with other teaching experiences, work with special needs groups can be frustrating. With dementia it is clearly unhelpful to focus on technical aspects, when the emotional content of the dance is manifestly important. But dancing in time to the music, and using the same steps as other dancers, is a form of conversation. How much more valuable and affirming it must be for people with dementia to communicate in this way, when their opportunities for meaningful contact are diminishing.

Another problematic issue was that of touch, a feature of most circle dances. What about those people with dementia whose earliest memories of touch were disturbing? Could circle dance revive painful memories of insecure attachment, or even of early abuse, violence and unpleasant sexual encounters, and further undermine fragile coping strategies? As the weeks went by it was clear that some people strongly resisted holding hands. If they inadvertently got involved they reacted with child-like intensity, withdrawing immediately. It would have been helpful to know what dance represented for each group member (pressure, sadness, romance?), and what feelings were engendered before and after dance experiences in their earlier lives. In the absence of such personal information we needed to be sensitive to displays of feeling which might suggest added vulnerability. It seemed important that care staff were able to cope with the associations which might be revealed, and with any sexual interest provoked by physical contact through dance. The quality of contact raised questions about the possibilities for reparative work with people with poor early attachments.[2] It was time for a wider search of the literature on therapeutic dance with this population, and for a more systematic attempt to establish the value of my own way of working.

Circle dance and dance movement therapy (DMT)

In the mid-1990s the literature on music therapy and dance with older people with or without dementia was sparse. In Britain, Ruth Bright's pioneering work on music therapy (Bright, 1997) and Stockley's on dance therapy (Stockley, 1992) offered support for this way of working. In North America there were more sources, like McLoskey's (1990) account of singing with terminally ill old people and Clair's (1996) publication. In terms of therapeutic dance with dementing people, the literature focused on ballroom dance, and its capacity to restore fading couple relationships. Circle dance could do more, I thought, since it evokes attachment experiences much more basic than that of adult partnership.

What is circle dance? This dance form developed out of traditional folk dance from around the world. A name associated with circle dance in Britain is that of Bernard Wosien, who reinterpreted traditional dance movements to enhance their symbolic and spiritual content. Wosien brought his style of dance to Findhorn in Scotland in the 1970s and since then it has become an increasingly popular form of community dance. Most circle dance teachers use a combination of traditional and modern music and choreographies, involving a variety of armholds and group formations (circles, lines, spirals, and so on). Circle dance brings together emotional, physical, cognitive and spiritual aspects of being. It emphasises relationship and group solidarity, but is also an intensely personal experience. People typically come to circle dance at a point of crisis or transition in their lives (Mulreany, 1994). This kind of dance is experienced as healing and life enhancing, as well as being fun and very good exercise. It brings heightened awareness of self and other, an opportunity to show feelings and make contact with other people in a safe environment.

Circle dance has therapeutic benefits noted in other kinds of dance. One is non-verbal communication or synchrony, which creates a powerful feeling of togetherness (Steiner, 1992; Feder and Feder, 1984). In a group setting this sense of harmony is even more profound. In circle dance, the introduction of individual variations disturbs that harmony, and has a noticeable effect on the group's energy.

Like other kinds of dance, circle dance can forge a sense of collective identity and belonging. Traditionally it has provided stability and support in times of personal, social and environmental change. Anthropologists have drawn attention to the use of community dance to help people cope with personal, social and environmental change, with difficult emotions like anger or grief, to contain anxieties, and to promote a sense of belonging (Hanna, 1988).

The most minimal of movements, such as gentle swaying from foot to foot, is a means of finding physical balance. In people with dementia this focusing on one's centre might help support the fragile inner balance which in the early

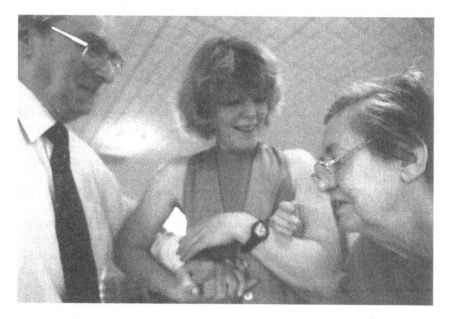

stages sufferers fight to retain. Similarly, rhythmic movement can allow the sense of self to be strengthened by emphasising contact with the ground, thus reaffirming our connectedness within ourselves and with the world through gravity (Steiner, 1992). In dementia, the sense of self is also strengthened by contact with other people. Holding and being held, the rythmic and repetitive rocking, swaying and walking are reminiscent of early attachment relationships.

One of the attractions of circle dance to vulnerable people is the belief that they will not have to expose themselves (King, 1996). The prescribed and patterned movements offer limited scope for individual expression. Rituals have a role in the alleviation of anxiety (Steiner, 1992). They allow a frightened person to hold on to the familiar in order to contain difficult feelings. In therapeutic circle dance, sessions are marked by a series of ritual events: the initial invitation to participate in the first dance, the teaching of steps and hand or armholds, the round of introductions after the first couple of dances, the reference to the origins and symbolism of the dances, and the expression of collective pleasure and mutual thanks at the end. Rituals are a feature of most formal gatherings of old people, expressing peer group solidarity and continuity through time (Jerrome, 1992). In therapeutic dance the rituals mark the boundary between the enfolding circle and the space outside it, which is dominated by different concerns.

Other boundaries are also asserted through the medium of the dance. Body boundaries, often distorted in psychotic people and others who cannot take their autonomy for granted, are assisted through physical touch. This works in dementia too, though, paradoxically, individuality in dementia, or person-hood, is affirmed by managing to do what the others do.

At first described as 'the music and movement lady' I came to be seen to be offering dance therapy to the people in the day centre. It was not dance therapy in the conventional sense, in which individual or group feelings are identified through spontaneous movements, or choreographed. With psycho-logically damaged children, for instance, the aim of dance therapy is devel-opment: to get them to do things they have never done before (Liebowitz, 1992; Stanton, 1992). With dementia, a progressive and irreversible disease, the aim is to slow the rate of decline, to help the individual make contact, to raise mood, to improve balance. In dance therapy with children and younger adults some caution might, as Steiner suggests, be advised in relation to aspects like touch and holding. Clients who did not get enough of these in early life might experience increased dependency. The dance therapy in such circumstances risks becoming an end in itself. With dementia, however, the aims are different. The transformative qualities of the dance lie in its capacity to hold and hold on to the person who is in the process of slipping away.

A research project

After the first series of dance sessions in 1996, and convinced by the evident enthusiam of the dancers and apparent benefits of the dance, it seemed important to evaluate the effects formally so that I could speak more convincingly about this kind of work, in a language fundholders might understand. With a manager from the day centre, who was also a trainee psychologist, I started to think about criteria for evaluation. We knew from the literature of dementia care that we were aiming for

- liveliness and stimulation, as opposed to apathy;
- sociability and other-orientation as opposed to withdrawn behaviour;
- attachment and warmth as opposed to hostility, coldness and disdain;
- emotional well-being, happiness and contentment as opposed to distress, confusion and parent-fixation;
- engagement (orientation to the here and now, enhanced short-term memory, attempts at communication) as opposed to disengagement.

Recent research (Bright, 1997; Donald and Hall, 1999; Violets, 1998) showed that after several dance sessions mental health improved, physical disabilities were less pronounced and general behavioural problems are diminished. Like other forms of pleasurable exercise, but with the addition of music, synchronised movement and physical contact, dance therapy could offer benefits in the form of

- improved fitness levels;
- mobility, balance and confidence in moving;

- improved circulation, which strengthens the immune system;
- a deeper level of relaxation;
- a general sense of well-being through the release of endorphins.

The evidence of existing research was that these effects lasted beyond the session, affecting mood and behaviour. The withdrawal into an isolated interior world, characteristic of dementia, was delayed. The heightened activity, the warmth of physical closeness, smiles and laughter generated by the dance, continued to influence behaviour. Non-physical benefits which had been identified included

- a chance to interact meaningfully with other older people and with carers, leading to improved relationships;
- a chance to express feelings, to revive memories of the self and share them;
- a chance to touch and be touched in comforting, socially acceptable ways, and to revive former social roles;
- a chance to make choices about involvement and contribute to the life of the group;
- exposure to new dance sequences and to familiar rhythms and steps which helps to maintain cognitive processes.

With these outcomes in mind we devised a set of affective, cognitive and behavioural measures to use in an evaluation of therapeutic circle dance. The overall design of the project reflected the holistic nature of the activity (therapeutic circle dance), the need of one of the researchers to meet the requirements of her postgraduate training in cognitive psychology, and my own years of experience as an academic social gerontologist with a background in social anthropology.

The study was conducted with older people in two day centres. There was an experimental group and a control group, sixteen people in each. The latter listened to music but did not dance. There were ten weekly dance sessions each lasting one hour. Tests were conducted before the first, after the fifth and after ten weeks. The three tests employed were the Mini-Mental State Examination (MMSE) as a measure of cognitive ability, the Clifton Assessment Procedure (behaviour rating section) and the Cornell depression scale (COR). Care staff were trained to administer the Clifton Assessment Procedure, while the researcher and two assistants administered the MMSE and COR. Care staff were also involved in qualitative assessments after each session, based on observation and interviews with the participants.[3]

The results were gratifying. Despite the brevity of the project there was a significant change in levels of engagement (communication, orientation to the here and now, short-term memory) among the dancers. Meaningful relationships had been formed involving heightened recognition and memory. There were also clear signs of a trend forming in physical abilities and mood-related behaviour. In short, the indications were that characteristics of dementia, such as memory loss and a decline in ability to complete every-day tasks and to communicate, were affected by the dance experience. After the ten weekly sessions the participants were more engaged, sociable, calm and happy. They also experienced increased energy and better physical control.

These positive outcomes were satisfying though we had been hampered by the small size of the groups and brevity of the study. Methodological prob-lems affected the statistical results particularly, with a failure to reach signifi-cance on some of the measures. Over a longer period, say six months, there might have been more profound change, delaying deterioration (though not reversing or halting it). Methodological problems such as small numbers and erratic participation were exacerbated by a lack of support from some staff at the day centre. It has to be said that staff resistance to the idea and reality of the dance sessions hindered the research process. Our results confirmed the importance of staff training and of attending to the needs of the caregivers, as well as those of the service users, during the dance sessions.

Training issues

Like the people with dementia, who bring with them early attachment experi-ences which shape their reactions to anxiety and insecurity, the staff have their own attachment histories. Often, early attachment experiences have been negative. People are often drawn to care work in the unconscious hope that their own attachment needs will be met. So for staff, too, inclusion in the circle can be a powerful and moving experience. Work with people with

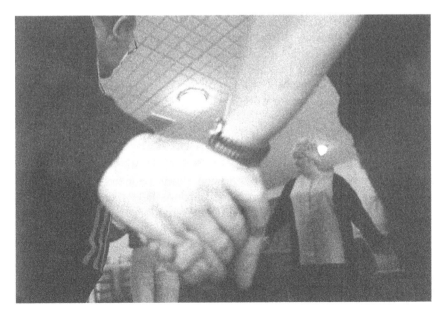

dementia is emotionally demanding, and therapeutic circle dance calls for particular abilities. It is now possible to identify specific requirements for staff to meet in order to be adequate facilitators. The following checklist is now offered in training workshops:

- openness to feelings, one's own and other people's;
- patience;
- the ability to stay with someone's expression of loss, insecurity, anxiety and pain;
- warmth;
- a sense of rhythm;
- physical strength and stamina.

Some preparation is necessary before beginning to dance with people with dementia. Staff need to experience the dance for themselves, to feel its power and emotional force. This serves as a reminder that if the dance can affect us, the caregivers, so profoundly, how much more powerful it might be with a person whose defences are limited.

Experience of working with practitioners has taught me that therapeutic circle dance is a particularly challenging type of intervention. As a result, staff practise various kinds of avoidance. The organisational setting, with adequate support, is critical for the success of therapeutic circle dance. If staff are not being held (metaphorically), it is unlikely that they will be able to offer this type of support to service users or expose themselves to such demands. People cannot easily allow themselves to recognise the attachment needs of others when their own are suppressed.

There is a need for briefing in advance of the work, in relation to attachment theory, the use of touch, and principles of validation. Workers need to have some idea of their own attachment issues and an awareness of personal boundaries. Feelings of anxiety aroused by close contact are allayed in staff who are aware of their own vulnerability in relation to the people they are caring for. Supervision is essential for staff support, a fact recognised by a leading exponent of this way of working, Marion Violets (Violets, 2001).

Practical guidelines

Sessions need to have a clear structure, with a beginning, middle and end. The opening talk and dance help confused people to ground themselves in the reality of their day. The break for refreshments allows them to talk and socialise. Rituals of closure (talking in turn about the experience of the session, expressions of thanks and farewells) allow the dancers to centre themselves again, to resurrect the defences temporarily lowered in the course of the session, and cope with the return to day-centre life.

Attention needs to be given to the physical setting: make it permanent, reduce distractions in the form of through-traffic and staff conversations. A notice might help other people to respect the space reserved for the dance. Suitable clothing and ventilation are important for physical comfort, as is the collection of appropriate medical information beforehand, and the adaptation of the dance movements (involving feet and legs, trunk, arms and hands, head and shoulders) to the physical capabilities of the dancers. Health and safety issues, and evermore stringent regulations, are increasingly pressing. We now recognise the need to divide the dancers into two groups – the chair-bound and more mobile – and treat them differently.[4] We have found that it works well to start with the full group doing seated dances adapted for the upper body only and with limited leg and foot movements, then when all are engaged to invite the more mobile to stand up and form a circle in the middle. The chair-bound people continue to take part in their own way, on the periphery.

The most important guidelines for would-be facilitators focus on communication as an essential part of therapeutic circle dance. In the course of the session the facilitator and care staff are active on all dimensions of interaction:

- *focusing* on the person;
- using *touch* for its own sake;
- communicating *verbally* whether or not we get a response;
- using *names*;
- becoming aware of *gaze* and *response*.

Conclusion

Used therapeutically, circle dance offers a chance to work holistically. Making use of touch, rhythm and movement, it builds meaningful relationships: between the leader and helpers and the dancers, and between the dancers themselves. This corresponds to the key principle of the new culture of dementia care, which is that the quality of the care relationship crucially affects the experience of the illness. In therapeutic circle dance the group experience is of paramount importance. The dance symbolises aspects of group life, something which is becoming increasingly tenuous for the old person with dementia. The individual is connected to others as a unique, sentient being with a life history, memories, skills and feeling.

The emphasis in therapeutic circle dance with dementia is on emotional bonds as a source of wholeness and personhood. The synergy of the dance – the sense of togetherness communicated non-verbally, that comes from shared rhythmic movements to emotionally evocative music – is the source of its power. This work is radical in both dementia care and in the world of circle dance. On both fronts it challenges conventional ideas of what is possible. In dementia care, where the medical model has been under siege for some time, the new paradigm of care offers fertile ground for the development of

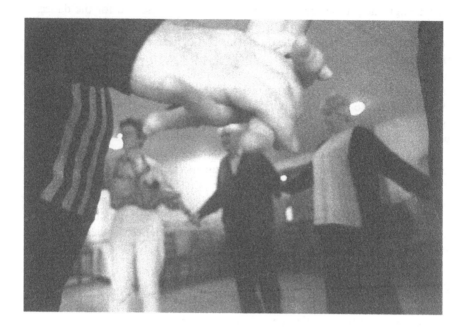

activities such as dance as a way of responding to psychosocial needs. In the world of circle dance there is relatively little work on dancing with people with special needs, though the transformative power of the dance is not a new idea. It has been known for some time that people discover or are typically drawn to circle dancing at times of emotional crisis or upheaval, at turning points when they are searching for new directions. Building on ancient community and spiritual traditions, modern circle dance has much more to offer them. The potential of folk dance as a non-threatening form of therapeutic movement in community mental health programmes has been recognised (Feder and Feder, 1984).

For healthy people, too, the circle dance experience goes on being emotionally powerful, providing opportunities for learning and personal development. One of the most humbling experiences of dancing with people with dementia is a sense of shared vulnerability. The healthy dancer also occasionally experiences being flooded with feeling – overwhelming sadness or anger or euphoria – apparently 'out of the blue'. Such feelings come from the experiential self, reached directly by the music and dance. This puts us, briefly and valuably, on the same emotional plane as the people we look after. Fortunately we are able to regain our composure, rely on our friends and fellow dancers to support us, and employ the strategies of the adapted self to return to normal life. Our clients cannot, but remain permanently exposed and vulnerable. This makes the ritual of closure at the end of a session particularly important as a way of returning to the here and now.

In working with the person with dementia we seem to gaze directly into the inner being, incapable of pretence or disguise. There is also a wealth of life experience there, most of it inaccessible. We do not know enough about the nature of being in dementia; like other one-way journeys no one returns to tell us what it is like. In the meantime we can do our best to assist the passage to an unknown future by providing meaningful activities like dance.

Notes

1 This chapter is an extended version of an article which originally appeared in the *Journal of Dementia Care*, 7(3) (1999).
2 I am grateful to the clinical psychologist Dr Fiona Goudie who offered some comments on this and other points.
3 For a more detailed discussion of the design and outcomes of the study, see Samantha Mansfield's MA thesis, 'An Evaluation of Therapeutic Circle Dance for Older People with Mental Health Needs', University of Sussex, 1999.
4 The last stage of the project involved collaboration with dance and movement teacher, Valerie Dawes.

References

Bright, R. (1992) 'Music therapy in the management of dementia', in G. Jones and B. Miesen (eds) *Caregiving in Dementia*, London: Routledge.
Bright, R. (1997) *Wholeness in Later Life*, London: Jessica Kingsley.
Clair, A. (1996) *Therapeutic Uses of Music with Older Adults*, New York: Health Professionals Press Inc.
Donald, J. and Hall, S. (1999) 'Dance: the getting there group', *Journal of Dementia Care* 7(3): 25–27.
Feder, E. and Feder, B. (1984) *The Expressive Arts Therapies: Art, Music and Dance as Psychotherapy*, N.J.: Prentice-Hall.
Goldsmith, M. (1996) *Hearing the Voice of People with Dementia*, London: Jessica Kingsley.
Gubrium, J. (1986) 'The social preservation of mind: the Alzheimer's disease experience', *Symbolic Interaction* 9(1): 37–51.
Hanna, J. (1988) *Dance and Stress*, New York: AMS Press.
Jerrome, D. (1992) *Good Company: An Anthropological Study of Old People in Groups*, Edinburgh: Edinburgh University Press.
Keady, J. (1997) 'Maintaining contact: a metaconcept to describe the dynamics of dementia', in M. Marshall (ed.) *State of the Art in Dementia Care*, London: Centre for Policy on Ageing.
Killick, J. (1994) *Please Give Me Back My Personality!*, Stirling: Dementia Services Development Centre.
Killick, J. (1998) 'It isn't fair when your heart wants to remember', in P. Schweitzer (ed.) *Reminiscence in Dementia Care*, London: Age Exchange.
King, J. (1996) 'My experience of dancing with special needs groups', in J. King (ed.) *The Dancing Circle*, Winchester: J. King.
Kitwood, T. (1997a) *Dementia Reconsidered: the Person Comes First*, Milton Keynes: Open University Press.

Kitwood, T. (1997b) 'The uniqueness of persons in dementia', in M. Marshall (ed.) *State of the Art in Dementia Care*, London: Centre for Policy on Ageing.

Kitwood, T. and Benson, S. (1997) *The New Culture of Dementia Care*, London: Hawker Publ.

Liebowitz, G.L. (1992) 'Individual dance movement therapy in a psychiatric setting' in H. Payne (ed.) *Dance Movement Therapy: Theory and Practice*, London: Routledge.

McLoskey, L. (1990) 'The silent heart sings', *Generations*, Winter.

Miesen, B. (1992) 'Attachment theory and dementia', in G. Jones and B. Miesen (eds) *Caregiving in Dementia*, London: Routledge.

Mills, M. (1998) *Narrative Identity and Dementia: A Study of Autobiographical Memories and Emotion*, Ashgate Press.

Mills, M.A., Coleman, P., Jerrome, D., Conroy, M.C., Meade, R. and Miesen, B.M. (1999) 'Changing patterns of dementia care: the influence of attachment theory in staff training' in J. Bornet, P. Chamberlayne and L. Chant (eds) *Reminiscence: Practice, Skills and Settings*. Dagenham, Centre for Biography in Social Policy (BISP), University of East London.

Mulreany, J. (1994) 'The Dance of Life', unpublished M.Sc. thesis, University of London.

Sinason, V. (1992) *Mental Handicap and the Human Condition*, London: Free Association Books.

Stanton, K. (1992) 'Imagery and metaphor in dance movement therapy', in H. Payne (ed.) *Dance Movement Therapy: Theory and Practice*, London: Routledge.

Steiner, M. (1992) 'Alternatives in psychiatry', in H. Payne (ed.) *Dance Movement Therapy: Theory and Practice*, London: Routledge.

Stockley, S. (1992) 'Older lives, older dances', in H. Payne (ed.) *Dance Movement Therapy: Theory and Practice*, London: Routledge.

Stokes, G. (1996) 'Challenging behaviour in dementia', in R. Woods (ed.) *Handbook of the Clinical Psychology of Ageing*, Chichester: John Wiley & Sons, Ltd.

Terry, P. (1997) *Counselling the Elderly and their Carers*, London: Macmillan.

Violets, M. (1998) 'We'll survive', unpublished paper.

Violets, M. (2001) 'We'll survive: an experiential view of DMT for people with dementia' in D. Aldridge (ed.) *Music Therapy in Dementia Care*, London: Jessica Kingsley.

Chapter 14

Nameless dread

A carer's story

Diane Waller

Introduction

It seems to be the case that many relatives of people with progressive illness, especially ones which involve dementia, feel a lot of guilt and anger at themselves for 'not being able to cope'. This can lead to physical or mental illness among carers, either during or after their relative's life, and the guilt for supposedly not caring enough can torment them indefinitely. With the emphasis now on thinking more positively about these illnesses and the quality of life which can be provided, there is a danger that carers may start to feel guilty about the negative feelings that they themselves experience or which they experienced while their relative was alive. It is clearly important that those closest to the sufferer maintain a hopeful, optimistic outlook,[1] yet this is extraordinarily difficult when the relatives are themselves trying to deal with their own grief and helplessness. In this last chapter, I share my own first-hand experience of progressive illness in the hope that it will strike some chords with others who have been in the same position and who have found the experience indescribably dreadful. At times my training as an art therapist and group analyst helped me to maintain some objectivity, at others it got in the way as I tried to 'hide' my feelings under a professional front. Art, in the form of conceptual sculptures, sometimes enabled me to put various experiences into a series of ironic, metaphorical processes, about which I will say more later.

Ten years ago I knew very little about Alzheimer's disease, and a bit more about Parkinson's. As far as other progressive illnesses were concerned, such as multiple sclerosis, motor neurone disease, Huntington's chorea, my knowledge was restricted to the experience of having friends become severely disabled (one later died), of supervising students working with patients having these illnesses, and in the last (Huntington's chorea), witnessing an old friend losing his ability as a musician and moving inevitably towards dementia. I recall the deterioration of a close colleague, an artist and teacher, whose loss of sight due to multiple sclerosis did not prevent him from making, through painting and drawing, an invaluable medical record of his experience before he weakened and died. The film *Hilary and Jackie* brought back the tragedy of this severe, relentless illness and how both an artist, and a musician (in the case of Jacqueline du Pré), had lost essential aspects of their identity as well as suffering the loss of their normal bodily functions. A friend, on the other hand, has had the disease for over twenty years and has some periods when she can almost forget she has it, and others when she is confined to a wheelchair, unable to speak. The nightmare for her is that she never knows when these periods will happen, so she and her family live in constant suspense. A psychiatrist colleague struggled with Parkinson's for many years before accepting retirement. He offered his experience of the disease in his book *Shadow over my Brain* (Todes, 1990). Supervising many students working with cancer patients in hospices taught me that even a single session of art therapy could provide a release for someone in the terminal stages of the illness, and that when all seemed quite hopeless it was worth giving just that bit extra to support the dying person in their journey.

Painful though all these experiences were and are, there was nothing to match the pain of watching my late husband, Dan, deteriorate through the stages of Parkinson's disease, to Lewy Body disease and losing his ability to communicate through a dementing process. Whether this was caused by the Lewy Body version of Parkinson's or whether Alzheimer's was another factor in this destructive combination, we shall never know. Our lives were changed completely: Dan's because he was suffering from a relentless progressive illness, retaining his awareness of this fact until he died, and myself for witnessing this, not wanting to accept it, becoming 'a carer' (a label I detest to this day though cannot think of a replacement) and engaging in a long battle on his behalf with the public health and social care services to preserve some quality of life for both of us – and, most importantly, to enable him to stay at home.

Dan also suffered from diabetes, so in the early stages of Parkinson's he volunteered to join a research project he had noticed in the *New Scientist* journal, run by Professor C. Mathias at the National Hospital, London, investigating possible links between diabetes and Parkinson's. For the duration of the project, Dan was monitored at the National and remained in touch up to a year before his death. He was due to be admitted for some reviews with the aim of trying to help his perceptual difficulties. Ironically, eighteen months after his death and two years from the initial invitation, I received a letter confirming his admission. Probably the most enduring benefit from the experience at the National was the attitude of Mathias himself, whose deep respect, concern and sense of humour, characterised the research interviews. Sadly, trips to London became more and more difficult as Dan's movement worsened, so the ordeal of getting to the National was too much. Depite the best efforts of the research team, it was clear that little could be done. We sensed the team drawing back, perhaps, unwillingly, 'giving up' on us. In these early stages his depression was severe – and who could be surprised as the future was uncompromisingly bleak. As Dan became more depressed and less interested in challenging his condition, I sought to read and understand about Parkinson's, and later about Lewy Body disease, and attended valuable research days organised by the Parkinson's Disease Society at Kings College. The medication, dopamine, could make a difference, but there was controversy about the side effects of another drug, selegelin, which Dan was also taking. Dopamine itself, when taken in the increasingly large doses needed to modify the movement difficulties, could cause hallucinations and frank psychotic episodes. Dan had bradykinesia and freezing rather than a tremor, so the dopamine did not help much. As the depression worsened, anti-depressants were added to the list, which already contained drugs to control his diabetes. I purchased a pill sorter, and every week carefully sorted morning, noon, evening and night pills, eventually adding antioxidants, New Zealand green mussel tablets (to help maintain joint movement), gingko biloba and aspirin to the little plastic containers.

Dan's psychiatrist at that time was very supportive of art therapy and arranged his attendance at regular individual art therapy sessions. It was a new departure for Dan, being 'on the other side' of art therapy, and it helped. Lurking always was the fact of deterioration, that 'this condition is organic'. My psychoanalytic training made me question such a cold fact. I think I held on to a belief that cells could be regenerated.

Perhaps one of the worst things was realising, from the moment of diagnosis of Parkinson's, that Dan had stopped being interested in living. He did, after all, know what the outcome would be, although mercifully not about the dementia at that stage. Whereas I was more inclined to maintain optimism that 'it doesn't have to be so bad'. I have always been a very optimistic person and proceed as if most problems can be solved, so I brought this attitude to something as devastating as Parkinson's. I now feel I may have been insensitive as it was not me having to deal with this catastrophic blow. Looking back, the optimism seems crazy; it was crazy, but perhaps it was the only thing which kept us both going. I fought against the futility and against a desire to give up myself. I know that Dan wanted to give up. He was a dancer and artist, very active, very articulate, loving to communicate. Above all he hated to be dependent and his worst fear was not to be able to be free to do what he wanted to do. An extrovert character, excellent athlete used to being a top performer, admired, he was reduced to shuffling with a stick, bent over, and eating, talking, dressing with extreme difficulty. A lover of good clothes, he was obliged to wear baggy track suits and easy-to-put-on items. Colleagues at the Sky Gym, our gym in Brighton, were outstandingly helpful: collecting him from home and taking him through exercises with light weights, stretching, and massage and, importantly, enabling him to feel part of the active world again. Never patronising nor irritable, Dave, Jenny and their team of instructors were invaluable support all through, giving practical, down-to-earth, genuine regard. It was such things that made the process bearable.

While Dan seemed to stop battling with his illness, and with his life, I seemed to be engaged in battles on all fronts. It was very difficult to find a place for him to be during the day, while I continued to work. I needed to work and wanted to. I was used to a full-time, demanding job involving patients and students, a lot of organising, professional activity, which I loved. As Dan's illness progressed it became difficult to maintain such a high level of commitment to so many different aspects of my work. When in London or abroad, when trusted carers were employed to stay with him at home, I was always anxious, waiting for a phone call to signal problems, and there were many. There were the occasions when he fell or some small misfortune occurred. The high quality of care needed drained all financial resources and he needed more company than could be provided at home. Eventually he was able to go to a day centre for people with physical difficulties, run by the social services. The environment was very pleasant, the food excellent and the young staff were helpful and considerate. The attenders were mainly elderly females, quiet and unassuming. Dan did not like it at all. He was popular with the clients but was challenging to some of the older female staff, hating to be pressured and cajoled. He did not enjoy any of the activities. Furthermore, he had no intention of even trying to! Compromise was not a word he understood. In the residential section, rooms could be booked for 'carer respite'. For a time this was a very good arrangement, but as Dan's mental state got worse it became difficult for the centre to provide for him. I was often telephoned following some altercation and summoned to collect this recalcitrant person. Rather like a mother telephoned when her child is misbehaving at school, I felt ashamed and irritated on both our behalfs. What was I supposed to do if a centre containing a large number of staff couldn't communicate with a non-aggressive but rather argumentative male! I felt very strongly that the older female staff really thought my role should be to stay at home and take care of 'the problem'. They never actually said so, and maybe they were not even conscious of it themselves, but looks and gestures and references to my 'important job' said in an ever-so-slightly sarcastic manner confirmed my view that feminism has a very long way to go and has not yet reached some south coast care centres!

I knew that, however difficult, and despite subtle (and not so subtle) suggestions, I should not give up my work, but try to modify the demanding schedule I'd maintained for many years and in which Dan had played an important role. When I had to go abroad for work it was possible for Dan to stay 'in respite' and, although expensive, I knew he was well cared for 24 hours a day. Going abroad was, I confess, a life-line, a bit of normality, an escape, an affirmation of identity. The fact that I was prepared to go abroad was greeted with incredulity and some sarcasm by some colleagues: so you can do that, then! I realised that the threat to the identity of a carer is a rarely acknowledged, or understood, phenomenon. A female carer's place should be in the home, or if not at home in her normal workplace! Or so it seemed.

Contemplating the pressures which abounded to 'give up and stay home', and perhaps 'keep the pain away from us', I felt that the Hindu practice of suttee, where the wife throws herself on the husband's funeral pyre, would not be such a strange concept for many people in England – although they would be horrified to hear this and I am sure would deny it vigorously. I feel shocked to have written it – but it is an attitude I have identified. I certainly feel that there is an aspect, maybe unconscious, in all of us, which would prefer sufferers from serious illness and their carers to hide away, and the carers too to sacrifice themselves to the cause of progressive illness. There is a shame attached to illness which lurks beneath our civilised veneer. In some of the carer groups I attended I was alarmed to see the extent to which some members, male and female, were bound to their relative, completely trapped within the notion that they were wholly responsible for that person. They had often retired, or had taken part-time work. They were exhausted and resigned to their lot. Sometimes I came away feeling fraudulent, angry and guilty that I was asking for so much help. Does facing a situation where you are helpless produce either extreme apathy or extreme energy in rapid succession, mirroring the worst aspects of Parkinson's? It is a question I often ask myself. Projective identification was certainly at work, and often. I was filled with rage one minute and sorrow the next; engaging in manic activity at one point and stunned into exhaustion at the next. Writing about it now seems like a dream, and I sometimes ask my friend and neighbour, did it really happen? She reminds me that it did.

There were so many incidents which reflected social ambivalence to the predicament of people with progressive and dementing illnesses. There are two which are firmly engraved on my mind: senior staff at the pleasant social services centre, where Dan had been going during the day and for respite, were becoming increasingly insistent that they could not meet his needs. However, finding a place that could was proving difficult. On Saturdays Dan used to come back in a taxi around 16.45, when I would be on my own with him until Monday. Later he was able to attend for several hours on Sunday. I was not able to leave him alone at all while he was at home, as he had several accidents, injuring himself by falling. He was perpetually restless, unable to sit, sleep, move, share what he was feeling, enjoy his food, and so on. Neither of us had any space or independence, which was extremely stressful for both. One Saturday, feeling very tired and down, I had a severe panic attack thinking of how I would manage this situation, and rang the centre, asking if he could stay a little longer as I was not feeling well. This was obviously a great irritation to the manager – though staff in the residential area 'upstairs' enjoyed Dan being there and did not have a problem. Feeling very put down, on top of everything else, made the panic worse, so I had the sense to request a visit from an emergency home-help later that evening. Knowing someone was coming allowed me to support Dan and to survive the panic attack. I had not had panic attacks before. It was time to take action. This was the point where I identified four young people skilled in working with people with serious illnesses. Some had already been coming for a few hours each week, working on shifts, being there when Dan returned and staying overnight, so I knew and trusted them. I had been up roughly six times a night for about a year by then, so their presence made an amazing difference. Had I not had regular full-time work it would have been impossible to pay these carers a decent rate. As it was, it took all my salary. But it was a question of survival. The positive side of this was that once in touch with the Alzheimer's Society in Brighton I was able to share all this with Neil McArthur who was an invaluable support, and with Wendy Lidster, my counsellor. Feeling alone – in fact, actually being alone because few friends and relatives could manage the pain and awfulness for very long – is something that most 'carers' report. I think also that it is very lonely being with someone you once shared everything with but can no longer communicate with. Another of the very positive things of this terrible period is the long-standing relationships formed with these young carers, of our chats sometimes late into the night and in the early morning when we were joined by my neighbour, and their excellent attitude to their work. We became a real team, which certainly lessened the anxiety and panic attacks as far as I was concerned and gave Dan a lot of young, stimulating company.

Indeed, if I were to be asked what was the most important aspect of the support I received it would be warm, non-judgemental attitudes combined with practical, down-to-earth help with everyday events – someone 'being there' to talk to.

The second memorable event in my life as a 'carer' was a 'case conference' called by the social services staff to discuss their wish to terminate Dan's attendance at the centre. They had been wanting to do this for some months. To be fair, the dementia was beginning to take hold and Dan could be 'difficult'. But he was never 'difficult' with certain staff and 'very difficult' with others. He had a loathing of being patronised and could sense it immediately. Whenever he felt patronised or pressured he became 'difficult'. Some of the young care staff at the centre said he was 'mischievous', and they liked being with him for his humour. Again, being fair, the centre was not equipped (through staff training) to help people with dementia or mental illness. Though I did observe some elderly women in the residential section who were decidedly 'demented'. A 'mischievous male' who will challenge attitudes is perhaps a different story . . . The social services staff were adamant that they could not have Dan there. It was agreed something else was needed. But what? At the end of the meeting, the decision was: 'stop this particular social services day care'. I asked: but what is the alternative, how long do we have to find another place, we have been trying but so far haven't found anywhere (which is clean, decent, with good staff and facilities)? The response was, it stops today. You can employ your carers. Or get an agency in. I was speechless and overwhelmed by panic. I had to go to work, I had to be with Dan, I couldn't manage Dan's relentless frustrating restlessness all day. It felt as if we were being punished. The meeting took place at a Brighton EMI hospital where we had occasionally had appointments. Dan was downstairs, in the hospital. My advocate Neil McArthur was also in shock at the sudden withdrawal of day care. There seemed to be no options – except the outrageous ward I had seen at the general hospital. Everyone left. I went downstairs in a state of near hysteria, Dan was wandering around looking anxious. I found the ward manager, and incoherently tried to explain what had happened. He was calm, incredulous, trying to fathom out how such a thing could happen. He reminded me that over three months before the case conference it had already been agreed that Dan was entitled to long-term health care (usually meaning residential care). He said, Dan can come here in the day, why not? And he will be used to us, he can have his own room, then if he stays over when you are away, he will feel at home. I'll sort it out . . . I knew Dan had met Kamal on several occasions and that he liked and respected him. Kamal behaved like a human being, concerned, ready to think of a way forward, not a cog in a system. It was a turning point, because although I found it intensely painful to acknowledge the worsening of Dan's physical condition and dementia, and very bad about myself for not being able to cope on my own at home, it was so reassuring to know that Dan (and I) would have the support of such rare people as Kamal and Neil. As to the social services staff, I was consumed with such hatred that I found it hard even to pass the building. Actually they were quite correct that they could not meet Dan's needs. With the packaging of people into categories, so prevalent in the social services, it was clear that Dan did not fit neatly into any of their categories. Therefore it was hard to meet his needs. Above all it was the smug and uncaring way with which these women delivered their sentence that got to me, the ready acceptance of the fact by the other staff present at the meeting and the 'washing of hands' of such a serious predicament by a group of supposedly caring professionals. Anyway, they were the targets for my rage for some time, before I brought my intellectual, rational self back into the frame and reminded myself that they were 'just part of the system, the pernicious system'. And they weren't confident enough to challenge it probably because they were women who had been used to being told what to do, not stepping out of line, fearful to do so. Faced with a woman who did challenge the system, they did not react like 'sisters' and feel glad and supported by this, but wanted to get rid of her – and have one less awkward relative to deal with.

Another difficult thing I found was relying on agencies. Once a week a night carer was paid for by social services, but they could only sanction this if an agency was used. Many of the young people sent by various agencies used over a two-year period were kind and responsible. However, they were not trained to work with people with the problems of moderate to severe dementia and they were paid atrocious rates. Some were in great need of support and counselling themselves. The better agencies tried to send the same person regularly, but this was hard because the turnover of young people was rapid and they sought better pay and conditions elsewhere. The agencies said they could only pay bad rates because they were paid so badly by the social services themselves. And so the system perpetuated itself. I tried hard to organise for the long-term health care we had been promised – which should have been paid through the NHS – to be implemented through the maintenance of my own team of carers and not through agencies or a residential care home. At the time, two years ago, this seemed a rather revolutionary idea. The notion was passed about from health to social services between January and July of 1998. It was, in fact, a much cheaper option for Dan to stay home with carers than to go into fully paid residential care. But it was not 'the norm', this being that the sick person went to residential care. After much hassling from myself, Neil, Kamal, and the consultant, the plan was on the verge of being put in place – but two days before the final planning meeting, Dan died, following a sudden severe infection and pneumonia. Perhaps some of those managers who would have had responsibility for sorting out this unusual package were relieved by the timing of Dan's death. There were others who were shocked and saddened. I like to think that things are now much more flexible concerning the framework for care, and know that several new and promising centres have opened in Brighton and Hove. I hope so. But then, I am an optimist.

From the small part that I have told of a very long story, it will come across that I remain very angry about the experience – and I am glad that I am. It is one example of muddled, over-bureaucratic and unnecessarily rigid procedures underpinned by the attitudes pointed out by several contributors to this book, in which the participants appear to lose their humanity. Frighteningly, a carer who is affected by the relentless and exhausting process of the illness can at times experience raging, destructive feelings for their sick relative and can hardly bear to be with them. Criticism, undermining or rejection, however slight, can be overwhelming as the carer struggles to maintain some normality. Nevertheless, I believe that I got more support and understanding than many people have done, or will have, and this was due to a few exceptional individuals. So I am angry rather than depressed and crushed, though it is true that for some time I lost all confidence in myself and had to struggle to regain it. The guilt remains.

Earlier I mentioned the role of art in helping to sort out the wildly mixed emotions experienced during this period, which were unfortunately compounded by changes in the workplace which caused further anguish during the two years prior to Dan's death, in perhaps the most difficult phase of his illness. In particular I am grateful to the late Ed Kienholz (1927–1994), a sculptor born in the USA to a farming family, who for several years lived and worked in Berlin. Kienholz was among a group of artists, including Richard Hamilton and Tom Wesselman, who created mixed-media tableaux. Kienholz could be considered as a 'pop' artist, but his subject matter dealt with the grimmer side of life – with issues such as war, abortion, alienation, prostitution and destitution. I came across his work in Amsterdam during the 1970s and was powerfully influenced by the impact of such works as 'The State Hospital' (1966), influenced by a period in which he worked in an asylum; 'The Art Show' (1963–77) in which one enters a room at a private view, complete with life-sized figures with tape recorders in their heads, endlessly muttering the banalities that are often heard on these occasions; and 'The Portable War Memorial' (1968), this last an ironical comment on the American involvement in Vietnam. The use of music in these tableaux was particularly effective. The seedy atmosphere, in which one feels and indeed is very much a voyeur, is replicated in a series of rooms based on the red-light district of Amsterdam – The Hoerengracht (1984–88). The claustrophobic existence of the prostitutes, who must wait for their clients, viewed like so many cattle in a market, is an extremely powerful and disturbing work. Ken Evans's chapter 'In the waiting room of the Grim Reaper' could inspire a Kienholz tableau. The ability of a sculptor to take apart the hypocrisy and idiocy of social life through these tableaux, where you, the viewer, can only watch, wait but not act, greatly impressed me. The fact that Kienholz had found inspiration for the objects used in his tableaux from the famous Berlin fleamarket was also exciting. I too scoured fleamarkets for 'useful' items, things which 'might come in handy'. Although my art school training was as a painter and printmaker, I had abandoned the flat image in favour of multi-media experiences, including movement and performance. After discovering Kienholz's work, I realised that I had often worked out problems by visualising how they might look if assembled in a series of human forms or objects, accompanied by music or sound. For example, on a trip to Berlin I was walking in a street in the old Jewish quarter of former East Berlin, before it was transformed into a trendy restaurant area. The notion of time passing and of the collision of incompatible cultures was very strong. I saw an old lady leaning out of a window, just watching her world change. It seemed as if she had been there for ever. Kienholz's tableau of an old lady in a room surrounded by her memories, 'The Wait' (1964–65), came into my mind. Then I thought of the old ladies I had seen in numerous residential care homes (as Ken Evans says, 'waiting'). Words came into my head 'Come on, Nelly!' Come on, come on . . . and how many times have I said that myself. Come on, Dan, come on . . . have your food, go to bed, get up, go to sleep, get dressed, go to the toilet . . . In a flash I had a visual image assembled from many actual images but distorted by time and by fear. While in Berlin I harassed my dear friend and colleague, Karin Dannecker, to help me assemble the objects for this tableau-to-be. Visits to the Brighton fleamarket secured the items that will go to make Nelly's surroundings and her clothes. Another idea, 'Once upon a Time, time, time . . .' came up when I started reminiscing about the past, hardly believing that the past existed, and being glad that then I did not know about the future. How futile it is to worry about the future. When does the past stop and the future begin? A monotonous voice, chanting these words accompanied by the ticking of dozens of clocks and watches, came into my head. For some months I collected old clocks and watches from fleamarkets, and they wait for their moment to be assembled. Perhaps they won't be assembled, and it doesn't matter as they have served a purpose. Berlin has been the stimulus for many such ideas, especially the chance happening on the major Kienholz retrospective in 1997. I dealt with a particularly upsetting incident in my workplace by assembling images and objects which went through several stages of transformation as 'Homage to Power and Control' before being transformed again into 'Second-Hand Rose meets Four-Star Fred for a Cup of Coffee' (Figure 1) (the last containing many verbal and visual references to the increasing absurdity of academic life with its emphasis on competition,

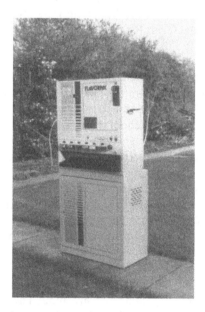

Figure 1 A drinks machine in a garden. This is one of the objects which made up the sculpture: Homage to Power and Control. It is an ordinary vending machine, old fashioned type, dispensing cheap, hot drinks. What is it doing in a garden? It looks as if it is waiting to be moved. It is a functional object which has no use where it stands. Later, it will be moved and will become part of another installation: Second Hand Rose meets Four Star Fred for a Cup of Coffee. The reader will have to imagine Rose and Fred as they have now left the scene. Rose has invited Fred to join her for a coffee and a chat. They have nothing in common except they are both outsiders in a system in which they struggle to find a role. Fred aspires to move from his Four Star status (one which only exists in his mind), but he is trapped by convention and desire (although if you ask him he doesn't really know what that means). Rose remains close to her roots and enjoys the game. Their story must wait to be told. In the meantime, the vending machine has found another useful role, dispensing drinks to men in a centre for the homeless. It will probably stay there.

league tables and with the still lamentable position of women in senior positions, for which I raided the vintage clothes store 'Garage' in Berlin and the Brighton fleamarket). I found it very pleasing and reassuring that Kienholz had found his inspiration in fleamarkets and similar places, and grateful for the example he provided. His work is not pleasant to view. Indeed it is deeply disturbing. For me, it was and is therapeutic to conceptualise certain events or combinations of events in sculptures, or tableaux, for which I have to seek out objects. Whether they ever get made or not seems unimportant. The searching for something (which may or may not end up in a sculpture) without knowing quite what helped me get through particularly terrible periods before and after Dan's death. I have observed that people with dementia are often searching too, maybe for their lost objects, lost parts of themselves.

Concerning Berlin, perhaps it is the extraordinary juxtaposition of so many nationalities, such histories, such opposing ways of life, such horrors, memories of violence by and to the city, and such vitality in the frenetic buildings that inspires. I always return shaken up and very thoughtful.

In getting back to the focus of this chapter, and in thinking about opposing cultures, it seems as if a change to the culture of dementia care urgently requires the proposed amalgamation of health and social services departments, for a start. Many of the problems I experienced were due to poor communication within and between services, those workers in the front-line trying their best to maintain a flagging system. Frequent cuts in resourcing made matters worse. But a lot of time and money was wasted in inefficient procedures. Most professionals are idealistic people, frustrated by their working conditions. I think everyone wanted to do their best but many were blocked.

Concluding thoughts

It is very hard to describe the thoughts and feelings that went through my mind during the worst phases of Dan's illness. I was constantly aware that if I was having difficulties winding my way through this maze of procedures when I am an articulate health professional, knowledgeable about the services, prepared to ask for what's needed, what must it be like for the often elderly relatives faced with the deterioration of their partner, or of those caring for parents, who have no idea of where to start and who may be fearful of professionals 'in authority'. We are a wealthy country with a long tradition of free health and social care. It is not true to say that we cannot afford provision for top-quality care. The subjugation of ethical and moral values to crude materialism is shameful. Witnessing young people homeless in the streets of affluent Brighton, child drug addicts unconscious in the gardens of the Pavilion, elderly people stupefied in front of a blurred television screen in some dismal private care home, is to me all part of the same picture – one where exploitation for profit is prevalent. Witness the disgraceful treatment of farm animals, treated as so many commodities, abused in a system where waste is a necessary feature. Since the first write up of this chapter we have experienced foot and mouth disease and the outrageous destruction of animals as if they were rubbish. This is a powerful symbol of a culture which disregards that which is no longer profitable. I am convinced that the myth that 'there is not enough' (money, resources) is one that is insufficiently challenged. It hits at the deepest human fear of being starved, left to die, so we must scrabble and fight each other for the crumbs. Whose interests does this serve? There is, in reality, plenty to go around. We are all part of 'the system' and, by challenging gross injustice, have the power to change it. Society doesn't exist outside ourselves so we can all try to make a difference even if it's a small one. Leaving it all to a fantasy 'them' is a cop-out.

Note

1 See Ridder *et al.* (2000). This article explores two issues involving the relationship between optimism and adaptation in chronically ill patients: (1) whether the impact of optimism on adjustment is disease-specific; (2) whether greater optimism produces better adjustment or whether, in contrast, a medium level of optimism plays a more adaptive role. The study recruited 166 patients with Parkinson's or multiple sclerosis. The study suggested that MS patients benefited more from optimism than PD patients and that in comparison with PD patients, optimism in MS patients does not necessarily promote avoidant and emotion-oriented coping. An important concluding comment was that: 'one should exercise caution about the assumed ever-present beneficial effect of optimism, regardless of the type of illness patients are dealing with' (p. 153).

References

Hopps, W. (1996) *Kienholz Retrospective*. Catalogue of the Retrospective exhibition of this artist's work in Whitney Museum of American Art, New York and the National Museum for Modern Art, Berlin. Prestel-Verlag, Mandlestrasze, Munich.

Ridder, D., Schreurs, K. and Bensing, J. (2000) The relative benefits of being optimistic: optimism as a coping resource in multiple sclerosis and Parkinson's disease, *British Journal of Health Psychology* 5: 141–155.

Todes, C. (1990) *The Shadow over my Brain: My Struggle with Parkinson's Disease*, Gloucs: Windrush.

Index

abandonment 2
abnormalities: early 29; gait 29; movement 30, 56; postural 33
absent-mindedness 97
absenteeism/absences 22, 83
abulia 30
abuse 7, 24, 42, 43, 86; early 172
accents 21
acceptance 89, 166, 167, 168
accomplishment 73
achievement 74, 84
acknowledgement 77, 115; verbal 80
acting out 40
action theories 23
activity disturbances 90
adaptation 166
adaptive cortical system 35
administrative functions 17, 18
admissions 20
aesthetic form 52
affection 43, 53, 55; concealed 53
ageing process 69
agencies 189–90
aggression 86, 128, 167; screening for 88
agitation 30, 80; screening for 88
Aids 101, 104
akathesia 30
akinesia 28, 30–1
alarm 31
alcohol abuse 57
Alzheimer's disease 1, 3, 9, 10, 47, 48, 68–83, 87, 123, 183, 184; art therapy and 52–5; mild to moderate, drugs available for 5; young sufferers 107–21
Alzheimer's Society 94–105, 122, 132, 143, 188
ambivalence 125, 126
Amsterdam 191
AN 1792 vaccine 5
analogies 31
anatomy 39
Anchor Trust 8
anger 28, 39, 44, 98, 128, 129, 145, 166, 172; transferred 110
anguish 19, 166
anthropology 92; social 176

anthroposophy 9
anti-depressants 185
antioxidants 185
anxiety 32, 34, 38, 41, 43, 57, 125, 126, 171, 188; alleviation of 174; aroused by close contact 178; catastrophic 6; clear signs of 7; constant 2; containing 173; control by breathing techniques 33; high 108, 113; learned 6; mirrored 112; reactions to 177; screening for 88; separation 112; unbearable 6
apathy 30, 31, 33, 57, 187; screening for 88
aphasia 169
appearance 24, 98; pride in 89
apprehension 103, 114, 151
'approach-avoid' style 169
archipallium 52
Ardis 143
Aricept 5, 96, 99–100, 109, 133, 144
artefacts 81
articulation 40
arts therapies 1–12; and Alzheimer's disease 52–5, 68–88; and Parkinson's disease 49–52
assessments 87, 88, 89, 91–2, 132; and confusion 92–3; observational 132
asylums 1, 191
ataxia 60
attachment 24, 173; childhood patterns 35; early 168, 174, 177; emotional 15; insecure 172; long-departed figures 167
Attachment Awareness and Dementia Care project 166
attachment theory 166, 178
attack 43
attention 31, 90; focused 116; lapses in 62; more focused span 109; sustained, measuring 124; visual selective 124; wandering 108, 113
attitudes 14, 142, 144, 190; accepting 162; bodily 38; care workers and managers 96; listener 33; 'positive' 123; public 84; sexual 91; social 17; staff 22, 126; warm, non-judgemental 188
Australia 9, 149, 150; see also Canberra; Melbourne

autocuing technique 146
automatism 157
autonomy 123, 174
autopsy 87
autosomal dominant disorder 56
avoidance 136
awareness 20, 33, 38, 39, 104, 142, 184; body
    44; dementia 96; full 65; impaired 62;
    metaphor 171; need for boundaries 36; new
    states of 47; of others 34; of personal
    boundaries 178; time 37; vague 166
awfulness 188

Bainbridge Cohen, Bonnie 34, 35
balance 35, 173–4, 175; difficulty maintaining
    61; impaired 28; lack of 29, 32; problems
    with 34; sense of 37
Balkwill, Midge 149
banal activity 141
Barthel Activities of Daily Living 124
basal ganglia 28, 56
beauty 48, 169
beds 86; blocking of 17, 88; filling 20; pressure
    to 'unblock' 88
Beeharee, Kamal 8, 10, 138–44, 189
BEHAVE!! AD (Behavioral Pathology in
    Alzheimer's Disease Rating Scale) 88
behaviour 61, 62, 63, 123; 'abnormal' 58, 91;
    aggressive 57, 59; altered 52; appropriate
    patterns established 36; attachment 166;
    atypical 91; bizarre 59; challenging 97;
    changes in 58, 60; contradictory 24;
    'delusion' 90; 'good' 89; inappropriate 53;
    mood-related 176; motor, aberrant 88;
    problems 57, 175; repeated 44; sexual 24–5;
    unreasonable 59; unusual 86, 91
being: different understanding of 34; difficulty
    of 1–12; doing and 49; emotional, physical,
    cognitive and spiritual aspects of 173;
    individual uniqueness of 167
belonging 83, 173
bereavement 42, 43, 135; powerful non-verbal
    acknowledgement of 77
Bergson, H. 4
Berlin 190–1, 192
Bion, W. 2, 4
Birmingham 146, 155
bitterness 145
blood pressure 41
boarding schools 18
bodily functions 184
body language 83, 99, 152–3
Bond–Lader Mood Scale 124
bonding 35
Booth, Dian 151
borderline personality disorders 36
Bosch, Hieronymus 19
boundaries 36, 43, 108, 118; awareness of the
    need for 36; body 174; personal, awareness
    of 178; redesigning 53; safe 113; space and
    time 40; time 125
bradykinesia 28, 29, 185

brain 28, 146, 147; activities associated with
    right side of 147; can no longer regulate
    body functions 112; descending extra
    pyramidal motor pathways 29; development
    35, 36; genetic systems that programme
    development 35; growing 35; instruction is
    imperfectly transferred 145; left analytical
    side of 147; most ancient part of 52;
    neuroreceptors 5; 'organic disorder' 1;
    reorganisation of structures 36; sensory
    information 35; visual image-making
    activates a part still intact 3; see also
    neurotransmitters
breakfast 22
breathing 33, 64
Breton dance 169
Bright, Ruth 171, 172, 173
Brighton and Hove 94–105, 123, 125,
    132, 138, 143, 144, 185, 188, 189, 190,
    193
Brighton Health Care Trust 122
British Association of Art Therapists 9
Brown, Melanie 146, 155
brutalising process 19
Bull, P. E. 33
bullying 21
Bunce, Jill 9
bureaucracies 16–17, 18

calligraphy 147
calm 74, 101, 112, 149, 150, 170, 177
Canberra 9, 148, 151, 157
cancer 10, 101, 103; patients in hospices 184
CAPE (Clifton Assessment Procedures for the
    Elderly) 124
care homes 112; converting bed-sits to 16;
    dementia sufferers abandoned to 15;
    hierarchies in 21; larger 87; main reason
    for admission of dementia sufferer 91;
    'placement' in 84; primarily businesses 17;
    problems relating to the quality of care
    that might be provided 87; route to 86;
    small 87; some owners reluctantly pay for
    occasional one-day training 22;
    unregistered 8
'care in the community' 9, 16
care managers 20, 87, 88, 89, 91; competing,
    behavior of 17; expected to apply rules
    impersonally 18
'care packages' 85
'care-plans' 16
'case conferences' 188–9
'cash-nexus' 17
Castorp, Hans 19
catatonia 31; symptoms of 30
central nervous system 56, 145
centres of excellence 96
cerebral cortex 36
cerebral lesions 52
certainty 51
Charcot, J. M. 30, 31
charity 143

chiaroscuro 49
choice 62, 82, 93, 123; freedom of 138; limited 108
chronic invalidating conditions 47–55
chronically mentally ill people 1, 144
Churchill Fellowship 9, 148
CIBI (Carers Impression Based Interview) 124
Clare, A. 173
claustrophobia 41, 113
cleanliness 24
Clifton Assessment Procedure 176
close relatives 91
closeness 166, 176
clothes 21
clues/clueing 146, 155
Clynes, Manfred 150
CMAI (Cohen–Mansfield Agitation Inventory) 88
cognition 37, 62, 123, 124, 136, 166, 167; capacities 37; deficits 74; difficulties 139; disability 30; impairments 10, 28, 32; malfunction 32; reduced capability 1; relationship between motion, emotion and 34; tests 132
cohesion 136
coldness 41
colours 49, 51, 117, 147, 149, 153, 154; related to emotional states 150
comfort 179
commitment 131, 186
communication 6, 52, 53, 58, 64, 65, 97, 123, 176, 179; about self 170; affected by ambivalence 125; attention to the subtleties of 2; difficulty with 136; flirtatious 135; illness gets in the way of 165; interactive 66; meaningful 2, 66; posture and 33–5; problems 28; severely impaired 61; see also non-verbal communication; verbal communication
compensation 52
completion 73, 75
complications 50
comprehension 28
concentration 57, 73, 113, 146; lapses in 62; limited 169
concentration camps 19
conductive educators 160
confabulation 23
confidence 85, 142; improvement in 44; lack of 34, 43; lost 126, 134, 135, 152, 190
confinement 113
conflicts 40; hidden or inner 82
confrontation 154
confusion 32, 59, 69, 70, 75, 80, 81, 92–3, 109; apparent 171; assessment and 92–3; major 103
connectedness 34, 174
connection 73
Conquest 9, 149, 155
consolidation 49
constancy 40

contact 34, 35, 85, 90, 174; close, anxiety aroused by 178; emotional and social 169; meaningful 172; physical 83, 172, 175
containers 77, 165
containment 53, 87, 88; suggested need for 131
contamination 143
contentment 153
continuity 82, 174
contortion 145
control 81, 82, 87, 158, 168; physical 177; unbearable thought of losing 112
control groups 122–37
conversations 23, 33, 170, 172; relaxed and rational 90; staff 178
conviction 80
co-ordination 61; co-ordination very disturbed 8; poor 169
coping strategies 172
Cormick, Moya 150
Cornell depression scale 176
cortex 32, 52
Cossio, Attilia 9, 149, 151
counselling 101, 144, 190
countertransference 113, 114; psychotic patients 4
CREATE (Center for Research Education, Artistic and Therapeutic Endeavours) 150
'creative accidents' 160
creative process 32–3
creativity 35, 146, 147, 151, 168; encouraging 149; help to stimulate 155; stimulated 40
Crickmay, C. 34
criticism 190
Crombie, Marjorie 159
crying 101
CSDD (Cornell Scale for Depression in Dementia) 124
cues/cueing 89, 155
cut-backs 86

dance 3–4, 11, 27–46, 108, 173–5; see also therapeutic circle dance
Dannecker, Karin 191
darkness 109, 113
day-care facilities 100, 108, 134, 186; dance 168–70; social services 134; sudden withdrawal of care 189
death 56, 74, 76, 79, 83, 86, 184, 190, 192; acknowledged 80; euphemism for 114; imminent 48
debility 31; physical 58
decision-making 37, 52, 64, 65, 82; encouraging 58
deep-breathing exercises 64
defacement 115
defences 49; healthy mechanisms 38; inappropriate 36, 43; limited 178; rigid 36
degeneration 1, 3, 50, 114, 120; cognitive 58; slowing down 52
dehydration 112
delusions 23, 57; screening for 88

dementia 7, 13, 14, 19, 27, 29, 40, 87, 122–37, 192; abandonment of sufferers to care homes 15; 'Alzheimerization' of 107; art therapy with older adults clinically diagnosed as having 68–83; assessing sufferers 90; assumption that sufferers have negligible personal insight 20; attention to psychological state of people with 8; chronic 112; common cause of 32; dance with people with 165–82; definition of 107; developing 30; diagnosis of 1, 84, 94, 133; drama is always present 4; early onset 100, 123, 138; features of 2; frontotemporal 147; GP has limited knowledge and understanding of 84; homely place for people with 142; knowledge that there is no cure 92; living with 94–106; medicalised 142; moderate 189–90; nature of 165–8; nursing and social care for sufferers 85; physical problems attached to 98; questions intended to reveal indications of 90; rights of those with 5–6; severe 54, 102; shaped by relationship 25; social and cultural backgrounds of sufferers 21; sociology of 13, 14; sufferers hospitalised for other injuries or conditions 88; symptoms of 23, 87; understanding people with 140; vulnerable patients 88; what the elderly sufferer gets in the way of care 17; worsening of 189; see also Alzheimer's; senile dementia
dementia praecox 107
denial 75, 79, 80, 81, 166
dependence 70, 87, 153, 175; levels of 17
depression 2, 28–33 passim, 47, 57, 97, 98, 123, 136, 145, 153, 166, 172; decreased levels 132; emergence of 1; exacerbated 112; life without 128; lifted 44; marked difference in levels of 124; need to alleviate 43; relieved 162; screening for 88; severe 105, 184–5; symptoms of 30; treatment of 49; underlying cause of 36
descriptions 40, 109
desires 47
despair 96, 123, 127, 128, 133; expressions of 167
deterioration 89, 185; delaying 177; rapid 112; relatives faced with 193
developmental stages 35, 36
DHSS (Department of Health and Social Security) 16
diabetes 184; drugs to control 185
diagnosis 87, 124; Alzheimer's 95; dementia 94, 97, 103, 105, 133; Parkinson's 145, 146, 148, 149, 153, 157, 185
dialogue 75, 116; group 109; limited 117
dignity 55, 128
disabling conditions 9
disappointment 90
disarray 113, 116
disarthria 56
discomfort 98

discoveries 51
discussion and evaluation 159, 160–1
disinhibition 86, 88, 91
disintegration 81, 167
disinterest 36
disorganisation 36
disorientation 27, 80, 82, 113
disrhythmia 56
disruption 82, 114
distraction 82
distress 19, 57, 166; cry of 167; equal for sufferers and carers 10
domesticity 127
doodling 149, 155
dopamine 5, 28, 100, 145, 185; death of cells 32; lack of 49
dramatherapy 4, 11
dread 109
dreams 55; continuous 32; premonitory 48
dressing 22
dribbling 28
drive 30
drug abuse/addiction 57, 143
drugs 49; anti-dementia 96; cancer 100; complications with 41; dyskinesia and 154; effectiveness of 30; excess of intake 32; hallucinations and 154; paranoia and 154; poor management 123; that do not cure 47
dullness 28
dysarthria 62
dysfunctional patterns 43
dyskinesia: drugs and 154; help to calm 154; violent 157
dysphoria 88

eating 28
education 22
education specialised 18
'efforts' 37
ego 8
embarrassment 28, 43
embryo research 5
EMI (elderly mentally ill) 17, 22, 23; homes 18; hospitals 189
emotions 3, 39, 50, 52, 53, 69; blocked 44; difficult 173; difficulty in expressing 28; embodied 68; exploration of 82; expression of 31, 35, 149, 123; felt but not expressed 28; important 82; inability to express 36; liberation of 48; listener 33; opportunity to understand own 40; processing 167; repeated discharging of 36; strong 143; tangled web of 91; ties with special persons 166; unfolding of 51; wildly mixed 190
empathy 7, 8, 10, 53, 162; ability to communicate 167
encouragement 148
energy 169, 173; lack of 31
enteritis 42
entrapment 153
escape 52
euphoria 88

evaluation 44
Evans, Ken 10, 11, 191
everyday tasks 177
Exelon 5
exercise classes 39
exhaustion 30; profound 31
existence 4; monotony of 16
expectations 89, 127; external 82
expertise 18
experts 85, 96
explanations 92
exploration 82, 156; of mortality 77, 79
expression: creative 58; non-verbal 71;
    symbolic 35; verbal 57; vocal 53; see also
    facial expressions
extrovert character 185
eye contact 154

facial expressions 41, 53, 59, 83; dullness of 31
failure 160; fear of 159
Falconhurst 141, 142
Falk, Barry 10, 133, 138
falls 22, 28, 29, 42, 86; fear of 34
familiarity 82
families 14–15, 16; formal and informal links
    between clients and 18
family history 41, 89
fantasies 22, 54, 162; healing 53; persecution
    54; stimulated 40
FAST (Functional Assessment Staging) 88
fear 34, 38, 127, 136, 143, 171; all-pervasive 2;
    descriptions of 109; figures who once
    allayed 166; lurking underneath 101;
    mirrored 112; terrible 2
feeble-mindedness 107
feedback 58, 64, 108, 132
feeding 57, 63
feelings 36, 39, 69; awareness of 39;
    communicating ideas and 116; difficult 174;
    embodied 68; exploration of 80, 82;
    important 82; liberation of 48; negative 183;
    painful 38; powerful 165; projected 101;
    raging, destructive 190; receiving of 103;
    responses and 33; underlying 38;
    undisguised 166
Fellini, F. 49
feminism 186
'festination' 30–1
Findhorn 173
fitness 27
fixed stare 28
fleamarkets 191, 192
floor work 34
flow 37, 38
focus 31
force 37
forgetfulness 24, 86; progressive 91
Foucault, Michel 19, 92
fragmentation 81
freedom 123, 142
freezing 29, 30, 103, 156, 157, 185
frontal lobe dysfunction 30, 32

frustration 39, 50, 98, 108, 113, 117, 123, 141,
    144, 153; expressions of 167; help to relieve
    139; intense 145; stress and 152; venting 85
functionalist theories 15
fund-raising 157–8
futility 114, 185

gait 28, 29
gastrostomy 63
gender roles 126
geriatric wards 104, 105
gerontology services 87
gestures 71, 186; body 53; facial 62; rhythmical
    51
goals 160
Goffman, Erving 18–19, 91
'good mother' 47
governments 17
GPs (General Practitioners) 84, 86–7, 105;
    cannot deal with dementia cases 88; do not
    like to admit to their ignorance 87; fear that
    they have around dementia 95; hardly aware
    of dementia 104
gravity 37
Greek dances 168
Greenfield, Susan 27
grief 2–3, 173; around impending sense of loss
    107; relatives trying to deal with their own
    183
'group cohesion' 125
group sessions 39–40, 43–4
group solidarity 173
guilt 43, 87, 91, 183, 190

habits 21, 24
Hagestuen, Ruth 150–1, 154, 155–6
hallucinations 109, 185; drugs and 154;
    screening for 88; visual 32, 54
Hamilton, Richard 190–1
Hampshire 166
handwriting 147
hardship 27
harmony 48, 173
health authorities 100
health care 122, 143; free 193; general
    improvements in 123; long-term 189;
    see also mental health
Health Services 84, 102
heart disease 10
heart failure 112
helplessness 133, 136; relatives trying to deal
    with their own 183
Henzell, J. 1
heredity 101
hierarchy 21
holding 175; maternal 120
holistic approach 150, 151
home-help 187–8
Home Life 16
homelessness 6, 16, 25, 33
HoNOS (Health of the Nation Outcome
    Scales) 88

'hopeless cases' 84
hopelessness 102, 104, 123, 140; realisation of 19
horror 104
hospices 101, 114; cancer patients in 184
'hospital discharges' 85
hospital wards 82, 88
hostility 131
housing 8
Hulme, Ursula 9, 149, 155
humanity 190
humiliations 1
humour 65, 188
Huntington's disease 1, 10, 183; definition and description 56–7; music therapy in 59–66
hypertension 29
hypotonia 29
hysteria 31; symptoms of 30

id 52
ideal type 18
identification 6, 7
identity 154; acquired 85; affirmation of 186; carer 186–7; collective 173; crisis of 97; 'death' 19; enhancement of sense of 52; loss of 34, 97, 102, 136, 184; previous 126; struggle with 69; work 129
images/imagery 13, 19, 31, 38, 68, 75–80 passim, 113, 135; body 32, 34; bright and active 117; complex 116; consistent 116–17; distorted by time and by fear 191; externalized 14; people shuffling and dribbling in geriatric wards 105; pleasure of creating 74; powerful 168; repetitive 71, 72–3, 117; subconscious 150; themes and 109; uncomfortable 14; uninhibited 109
imagination 52, 76, 78, 79, 145, 146, 148, 149; 'hallucinatory' 109; opportunity to stimulate 150
impatience 30
impotence 49, 52, 136
improvisation 34, 60; 'goodbye' 65; instrumental 58, 59
impulse 31
inadequacy 52; deep sense of 47
incompetence 6, 23, 24
incontinence 89, 98, 99
independence 113, 115, 138; loss of 27
'independent providers' 86
individuality 175
industrial therapy 139
infantilisation 140
infection 112; severe 190
information: processing 61; retrieval 57
inherited illness 95
initiation 35, 57, 62; poor 61
inner world 73; withdrawal to 166
insanity 95, 107
insecurity 51, 152; reactions to 177
insights 20, 40, 57, 83, 89, 102; 'personal' 92

inspection issues 17
inspiration 146, 191
institutional incompetence 85
institutionalisation 112
integration 38; sensory 35
intellectual faculties 50
intelligence insult 141
intensity 37
interactions 18, 65, 131, 179; discrete 21–2; fragmentary 23; of self and others 37; see also social interactions
interference 36
international corporations 17
interpretation 39, 171
interruptions 108, 113
intimacy 35, 47, 131
intuition 48
IQ tests 91
irritability/irritation 57, 129, 187
isolation 29; emotional 69; increasing 59, 60; social 49–50, 123
Italy 148, 149; see also Milan; Monza; Turin

Jerrome, Dorothy 9
John Paul II, Pope 104
Johnson, Edward 3
jolliness 101
Joseph, B. 31
judgement 1, 122

Kafka, Franz 19
Kestenberg, J. 36
Kienholz, Ed 190–1, 192
Killick, J. 171
Killick, K. 6
kin 15
Kitwood, Tom 5, 7–8, 10, 166
Klein, Melanie 6
knowing 83; lack of 98
Kuhn, Thomas 92

Laban, R. 37
labels 104, 107
lability 37, 59
Laing, R. D. 23, 92
Lakke, Johannes 146, 151, 156, 157
Lamb, Warren 37
language 1, 49, 51, 52, 98, 122; abilities reflected in use of 169; common 5; creative use of 171; improvement in 53; less formal 78; limited 8; loss of functions 147; lost capacity to express through 165; professional 17; simple and affectionate 53
laughter 176
L-Dopa 5, 98, 100
league tables 88
learning: disabilities/difficulties 138, 139; interpersonal 49
Lees, A. J. 30, 31
legislation 16
leisure activity 64
lethargy 114, 153

Lewes 100
Lewy bodies 28, 32, 104, 184, 185
liberation 47
libido, loss of 27
Lidster, Wendy 188
literature 92; French 102
local authorities: assessment procedures 84–5;
    capacity to provide services for dementia
    sufferers 86; care managers working for 84;
    deals done between 17; housing
    departments 88; policies for residential
    care 16
London, National Hospital 184
loneliness 2
losses 1, 38, 42, 43, 44, 101, 123, 166, 169, 171,
    172; ability to express 144; aggression and
    anger 128; capacity to find words 141;
    considerable 69; deep sense of 47; difficult
    to come to terms with 80; faculties 5; grief
    around impending sense of 107; multiple 40,
    68; painful experience of 167; powerful
    indications of 127; reminders 131; strong
    theme of 136; unresolved 40
love 25, 167
Luria, A. R. 102

McArthur, Neil 5, 8, 10, 123, 188, 189
McInally, Finlay 10, 123, 124, 131, 134–6
McIntosh, G. C. 151
McLoskey, L. 173
madness 4, 5, 23, 112; marked by failure or
    loss of mental powers 107; non-sociological
    theme of 22; 'official' measurement of 91
Magee, Wendy L. 10
Maiorana, Wendy 156, 157
malfunction: cognitive 32; visual and
    proprioceptive 29
malnutrition 112
mania 57
manners 21
manual ability 52
Margate 149
marital breakdown 59, 90
marital therapy 39
marketplace 17
Marsden, C. D. 30, 32
Marx, K. 17
mask-like expression/face 149, 169
mastery 74
materialism 193
Mathias, C. 184
Mead, George 23
meals 22
meaning 23, 64; personal 171; shared 23
medication 11, 24, 29, 145, 149, 150;
    administration of 22; changes to 41;
    dependence on 27; ineffective 30; PD 147
Melbourne 146
memory 1, 35, 41, 54, 55, 62, 75, 122; dementia
    strips 98–9; difficulty with 136; fond and
    treasured 74; holding 118; impairment of
    30, 60, 75; long-term 23; losing 101; muted

167; old and well-established traces 172;
    problems 138; recaptured 73; see also
    memory loss; short-term memory
memory loss 69, 70–1, 72, 80, 177; apparent
    81; escorting the older person with 83;
    severe 97
mental faculties 145
mental handicap 2–3, 4, 104, 139; severe 1
mental health 91–2, 141, 165, 168; assessment
    in 91; care 87; improved 175; issues 88;
    nursing 138; people with problems who can
    express themselves 141; training of staff in
    141
mental hospitals 18
mental illness 92, 102, 188; among carers 183;
    general culture of confusion about 84;
    severe 141; terms for 104
mental state 148, 186; variations in 151
metaphors 31, 32, 38, 47; artistic 48; awareness
    of 171; body 34, 40; for fears and anxieties
    109
Miesen, Bère M. L. 5, 166–7
Milan 9, 49, 52, 149
military establishments/institutions 18, 19, 21
Miller, Bruce L. 147
Mills, C. Wright 13
mind 3, 54, 103
Minneapolis 150
mirroring 118
misdiagnosis 123
misunderstanding 48
mixed messages 33
MMSE (Mini-Mental State Examination)
    88–9, 124, 176
mobility 29, 33, 34, 37; loss of 27
modernisation 15
Mohammed Ali 104
monasteries 18
money-making 16
Montagu, A. 35
Monza 49, 52, 149–50
mood 144, 161, 169, 175, 176; changes 32;
    improved 132; posture might be altered by
    33; sullen 24; swings 32
mortality 69; unconscious exploration of 77,
    79
motion 37; lack of 31
motivation 28, 31; lack of 43
motor functions 28–30; fluctuations 146; skills
    58, 170
motor neurone disease 10, 183
mourning 78
mouth 169
Movement Disorder Clinic 146
movements 3–4, 9, 19, 30–1, 37–8, 179; central
    component for 33; choreic 56, 58, 59, 61, 64;
    clumsy and jerky 60; constant 63;
    controlled, loss of 145; early memories of
    172; exploring movement in a way which
    extends a patients range of 34–5;
    involuntary 64; kick-starting 155–7; large
    58, 64; minimal 42, 58, 64, 65; muscle

groups work together to support 34; music and 3–4; 'paradoxical' 39; prescribed and patterned 174; repeated 44; rhythmic 174; rigid 58, 64, 65; social interaction unconscious 33; spontaneous 175; struggle to control 145; swaying 60; uncontrolled voluntary 58; voluntary, abnormality of 56; worsened 184; *see also* akinesia; bradykinesia; motor functions
multiple sclerosis 9, 10, 183
Multiple Sclerosis Society 157
multi-infarct 104, 123
multi-media experiences 191
Murdoch, Iris 104
muscles 39; contracted 36; facial 28; finger 147; groups work together to support movement 34; jaw 28; lost control over 169; speech 29
musculoskeletal disorders 29
music and movement 3–4, 11
music therapy 10, 56–67, 148, 151, 154, 155, 160, 162, 168, 169, 171, 172, 173, 175; as part of a treatment programme 58–9; literature review 57–8
muteness 123

nasogastric feeding 63
National Institute of Conductive Education 155
Nazi regime 9
negativity 96, 102, 127, 177
neglect 86
neuropsychiatric inventory 88
neurosis 30, 31
neurotransmitters 28; deficiency of 30; fluctuating levels 32; *see also* noradrenaline; serotonin
New Scientist 184
NHS (National Health Service) 68, 88, 123, 190; document, *Making a Difference* 105; pay scales 133
'no hope' culture 8
non-pharmacological treatments 52
'non-productive' people 8
non-verbal communication 33, 167, 173; alternative 81; powerful acknowledgement of bereavement 77
noradrenaline 30, 32
normality 186, 190
norms 15
nuclear family 15
'nurses' 8, 19; *see also* RMNs
nursing homes: ill-equipped to provide spaces where creative activity can take place 4; privately registered 97; residents 166

objectivity 183
objects 7, 191; fast-moving 39; lost 192
observation 23, 37, 38, 124
occupational differences 21
old people's homes 82
openness 141, 142

opposites 31
optimism 185
orderliness 21
organic problems 1, 98
organisation 35
orientation 37, 90, 92, 176; reality 167
originality 145, 146
outreach 142, 143

pain 44, 51, 55, 154, 172, 184, 188; ability to express 144
Painting with Parkinson's 148, 157–60, 161, 162–3
pairing 77, 79
panic 6, 19, 113
panic attacks 187, 188
'paradigmatic shifts' 92
paranoia 154
parents: caring for 193; fixation 166–7
Parkinson, J. 31
Parkinsonism 28, 31, 156
Parkinson's disease 1, 9, 10, 47, 98, 100, 104, 123, 129, 145–64, 183, 184, 185; art therapy 49–52; case study 40–4; dance movement therapy 27–46; developmental movement 35–6; developments in the treatment of 5; diagnosis of 105; 'freezing' element of 103; groups 39–40, 43–4; idiopathic 28; motor function 28–30; movement analysis 37–8; movement in 30–1; postural changes in 32–5; psychiatric features of 32
Parkinson's Society 39, 104, 105, 148, 161, 185
Parsons, T. 15
passion 25
passivity 31
patient 'throughput' 88
Peake, Mervyn 146
peer group solidarity 174
perceptions 16, 21, 50, 51; inadequate 35; sensation and 99; very disturbed 8
perceptual skills 169
persecution fantasies 54
person-centred care approach 97, 104
personal hygiene 22
personality 38, 44, 65; affected 98; changes 57; imbalances 37; pre-morbid 31; traits of 36, 44
Peto, Andras 155
philanthropic organisations 158
philosophy 92
physical difficulties/disabilities 10, 148, 175
physiology 34
pictures 5
Pillgrab, Elisabeth 151
play 40
pleasure 47, 48, 50–5 *passim*, 62, 63, 170; collective 174; of creating images 74
pneumonia 190
poems 151, 155, 158–9
'pointlessness' 127
politics 143
Porter, Roy 92

'positive regard' 43
posture 28; abnormal 33; communication and
    33–5; flexed 29; positive 167; therapeutic
    process and 32–3
potentialities 53
powerlessness 129
PPP (Private Patient Plan) Health Care Trust
    122, 133
Pratt, John 162–3
Pré, Jacqueline du 184
preoccupations 116
pressure 172
pretence 166
prisons 18, 19, 140, 142, 143
privacy 82
problem-solving 57
procedures 193; inefficient 192
profit 16, 17, 86, 105; exploitation for 193
prognosis 104
progressive illness 1, 7, 11, 187; couples
    desperately trying to cope with 8; features of
    2; organic 3; staff caring for the sufferer 6;
    see also Alzheimer's; Huntington's; motor
    neurone; multiple sclerosis; Parkinson's
projective identification 6, 187; staff in
    institutions subject to 7
prostitution 191
protection 80, 140
psychiatric disorders 57
psychiatry 124
psychoanalysis 2
psychodynamic therapy: few patients with
    progressive illness currently have access to 4;
    persons traditionally excluded from 2
psychological problems 98
psychology 87, 91, 124; cognitive 176;
    experimental 10, 133
psychometric tests 100
psychosis 2, 4, 32, 98; see also psychotic
    patients
psychosomatic illness 105
psychotherapeutic process 36, 37
psychotic patients 174, 185; chronically ill 1;
    countertransference with 4
public opinion 17
'pulsion' 30
punishment and control 19
purpose 69

quality of life 29, 96, 101, 134, 151
quietness 74

rage 6, 144, 167
Reagan, Ronald 104
reality 23, 92, 177; concerning dementia
    sufferers 85; external or shared 120; inner
    120; meaning of 23; protection from 80;
    psychic 120; struggling with 80
Reality Orientation Assessment Lists 88
reasoning 1, 23, 122
reassurance 83
rebirth 74

reception 18–19
recognition 134, 176
redundancy 81
referral 85, 88
reflections 51
reflexes 29
refuge 115, 117
Registered Homes Act (1984) 16
registration 17, 22
regulations 16–17; stringent 179
rehabilitation 49
reintegration 83
rejection 41, 190; psychological 43
relationships 18, 36, 97, 123; bleak 25; body
    33; colour 156; conjugal 91; couple, fading
    173; defined 21; differences 21; earliest 15;
    emotional 35; family 32, 43, 58; group 33;
    improved 176; intimate 35; long-standing
    188; loss of 136; meaningful 53, 58; new 53;
    personal 17, 92; social 20; space 156;
    strained 32; unconscious 37
relaxation 31, 57, 150
remembering 62
reminiscence 66
Reminyl 5
renewal 74
repetition 31
residential homes 16, 95–6, 97, 190, 191;
    characteristics 18; managers of 18; quality
    of care 105; relationships between dementia
    sufferers in 20; residents' rooms 20;
    stretched by staff shortages 19
resignation 140
resistance 19, 31, 36, 108, 177
Resnik, Salomon 4
responses: absence of 62; caring 110; delayed
    62, 63; feelings and 33; motor 38; sad 110;
    verbal 116
restlessness 30, 80, 189
retirement 81, 97, 127, 129, 184
rhythm 51, 155; communicating through 168;
    early memories of 172
rigidity 29, 49, 56
risk-matrix 85, 91
ritual 73, 174, 178; shared 5
RMNs (registered mental nurses) 22, 87,
    100
roles 144; gender 126; social 19, 127;
    specialised 18
romance 172
Rotary 157
routines 22
rules 131
Rusted, Jennifer 123, 133

Sacks, Oliver 31, 102, 156
sadness 65, 90, 101, 110, 123, 166, 169, 172
safety 22, 167
saliva 28
satisfaction 117
Schaverien, J. 5
schizophrenia 107, 165, 169

Schore, A. N. 36
Scotland 173
Scott, J. P. 36
secondary illness 56, 123
security 40, 166; cry for 167
Segal, H. 6
selegelin 185
self 4, 7, 170; adapted 166; body is central to an understanding of 33; communications about 170; creative 49; deeper knowledge of 48; depressed 112; experiential 166; fragile 52; gradual deconstruction of 52; greater sense of 34; interactions of others and 37; mortification of 19; projection of parts into an object 6; symbol of 113; true 166; see also sense of self
self-awareness 34, 40, 173; stronger 53
self-belief 152
self-consciousness 43, 161
self-esteem 19, 42, 154; improvement of 49; increased 162; low 27; strengthened 52
self-evaluation 160
self-expression 161
self-regard 43
self-sufficiency 49, 50
self-therapy 148
senile dementia 1, 95, 104, 107, 139
sensation 98-9
sense of self 118; diminishing 19; made desolate 115; re-established 120; strengthened 174; way to reinforce 5
sensitivity 48, 50
sensory organisation 35
separation 24, 77, 79, 92; move towards 115
separation anxiety 112
sequencing 35
serious disabilities 29
serotonin 30, 32
sexual issues: disinhibition 86, 91; inappropriateness 57; loss of potency 129; loss of sexuality 136; unpleasant encounters 172
Shamash, Kim 123, 133
shame 2
shapes 147
Sheppard, Linda 123, 124
short-term memory 23, 90, 176; impaired 172; loss of 27, 71; problems with 59
shouting 167
shuffling 29, 105
side effects 185
sight 154
signals: non-verbal 7; social 21
signs 28, 49
silence 78
silly games 141
Simon, Rita 9, 148, 149, 156
Sinason, Valerie 2-3, 4
sitting 33
Skailes, C. 1

skin 35
Slavek, Peter 19
sleep disturbances 31
smells 20
smiles 176
Smith, E. 30
social change 17
social class 21
social conditioning 98
social differences 21
social environment 35-6
social institutions 15
social interactions 9, 21, 23; facilitating 22; importance of 36; promoting 144
Social Services 84, 86, 88, 95, 188, 190; care managers 17-18, 87, 89; day centres 134; Inspectorate 16; packaging of people into categories prevalent in 189; proposed amalgamation of health and 192; referral to 85; tussle between health care and 143
social skills 170; poor 62
social workers 84, 87, 91
socialisation 4, 35, 58; primary 15
sociology 16, 18, 20, 21, 87; bureaucratic ethos of 13; of dementia 13, 14
solitude 115
sound 154
South Downs Health Trust 100
space 4, 34, 37, 78, 148; active, symbolic 117; free from disturbance 115; holding 116-20; internal 115; narrowed sense of 112-14; private 20; safe 40, 108-9; time boundaries and 40
spatial orientation 35
Special Needs grant 148
speech 2, 29, 59; difficulty with 40, 57, 58; dysrhythmic and dysarthric 56; flighty and seemingly muddled 116; functional 62; muscles of 29; nearly impossible to understand 62; poorly articulated 61; severely impaired 63; slowed 30; slurred 60; unusually creative 171
speech therapy 39, 150
sponsors 157-8
spontaneity 135; loss of 57; marked lack of 61
'Spring' (Parkinson's disease research group) 27
stability 33, 37, 38, 173; lack of 33
staff turnover 22, 190
Standal, S. 43
standing 33, 34
staring eyes 28, 169
Steiner, Rudolf 149-50, 175
Steiner schools 158
Stelazine 24
stiff joints 40
stigma 57, 144
stillness 74
stimulation 50
stimulus 36

Stockley, S. 173
stories 40, 151
stress 32, 42, 123, 142; frustration and 152;
    safe environment to alleviate 43
strokes 1, 9, 10, 48
Struthers Parkinson's Center 150–1
stupidity 2–3
subconscious 149
substantia nigra 28
suffering 27, 140
suicidal tendencies 57
superego 52
supervision 178; important for care workers to
    have 101–2
support groups 42, 101, 149
surgery 145
Surrey 149
surveillance 25
survival 2, 8, 188
suspense 184
suttee 187
swallowing 28, 57
symbols 5, 35, 47, 126–7, 129, 174; intricate
    assemblage of 109; of self 113
symptoms 28, 29, 35, 44, 49, 147; behavioural
    62; cognitive 57; considered to define
    dementia 87; dementia 112; distressing 145;
    Huntington's 56, 62; 'living death' 30;
    motor 30, 31, 32; Parkinson's 41, 145, 151,
    156, 160, 162; physical 30, 38, 44, 59;
    psychological 30; psychotic 32;
    schizophrenic 57
synchrony 173
Szasz, Thomas 92

tactile experience 35
t'ai chi 151
talking 30
Tavistock Clinic 2, 138
tension 33, 134, 154; arms rigid with 169;
    inner 30
terror 2, 103
Thant, M. H. 151
therapeutic circle dance 9, 165–82
therapeutic culture 141
thinking 3, 4, 30, 38; rational 48
Thomson, Martina 150
thoughts: creative 52; horrible 110;
    important, exploration of 82; liberation of
    48; muddled 113; slowness of 30, 32;
    unfolding of 51; uninhibited 109;
    'wandering' 4
ties 80
time 37, 40, 141; awareness of 37; consistent
    82; disordered individuals 169; passing of 4;
    uninterrupted 148
Tingey, Nancy 9
tiredness 31; extreme 30
Todd, M. E. 38
Todes, C. 31
togetherness 173
toileting problems 98

torment 2, 103, 183
total institutions 18, 91
touch 2, 35, 154, 155, 167, 172, 174, 175, 178;
    communicating through 168
Towner Club 103, 138, 140–1, 142, 143
training 86, 105, 141, 144; awareness 96;
    in group dynamics 160; issues 177–8;
    managers and care workers 96–7;
    specialised 18
traits 44; fixed 36
transformations 69
traumas 27, 43, 143, 148; emotional 36, 40
tremors 28, 29, 49, 145; exacerbated 38; help
    to calm 154; settled when drawing 156;
    stubborn 157; violent 31
triggers 146, 160
trust 82
Tufnell, M. 34
Turin 51
turmoil 94; emotional 59; inner 7
turn-taking activities 60, 61, 63
Tyler, John 10

uncertainty 27, 96
unconscious 52, 76, 82
understanding 8, 138, 140, 141; communal 5
unease 50, 55; general public 91
uniqueness 53
United States of America 148
University College London 11
unreality 22
urgency 30

vaccines 5
validation 178
values 49, 84; ethical and moral 193; social 14,
    15, 92; staff 22
verbal communication 1, 58, 167, 169;
    impaired 71; limited 60; not possible 35;
    unconsciously influenced by postural
    changes in others 33
verbal process 38–9, 40
verbalisations 62, 81
Vietnam 191
violence 172; memories of 192
Violets, Marion 178
visualisation 34; guided 150
vitality 31
voluntary sector 143
vulnerability 71, 134, 172

waiting 14; endless and purposeless 22
walking 30, 33, 59, 160; absence of swing in
    the arms 31; hesitant 29
Waller, Dan 144, 184–90, 191, 192, 193
Waller, Diane 6, 160
wandering 23, 86; night-time 98
ward managers 142, 189
'wards for the elderly' 9
washing 22
Weber, Max 18
weight 37

welfare 69
well-being 38, 42, 44, 47; physical 69; sensitive
    concern for 80; strengthened 52
Wesselman, Tom 191
Winnicott, D. W. 38, 118–20
withdrawal 30, 97, 166; need to alleviate 43;
    social 59

Wood, C. J. 1
Wosien, Bernard 173
writing 2

Yalom, I. 125, 133
yoga 149, 151
Young, R. 31

Milton Keynes UK
Ingram Content Group UK Ltd.
UKHW040100071024
449327UK00019B/692